MW01233789

EXTREME WEIGHT LOSS HYPNOSIS:

2 books in 1:

Extreme weight loss hypnosis for women & Gastric Band Hypnosis. Stop Sugar Cravings, Emotional Eating and Change your Food Habits. Burn Fat Rapid & Natural.

This Book Includes

BOOK 1: 16 (FIRST PAGE)

EXTREME WEIGHT LOSS HYPNOSIS FOR WOMEN

Reprogram Your Subconscious To Lose Weight Without Effort Control Your Mind And Change Your Food Habits Stop Emotional Eating And Increase Your Wellbeing

BOOK 2: 208 (FIRST PAGE)

GASTRIC BAND HYPNOSIS EXTREME WEIGHT LOSS

Discover the Powerful Hypnotic Effect of Positive Affirmations. Control Sugar Cravings and Weight Gain with the Power of Meditation and Mindset Change

© Copyright 2021 - all rights reserved.

EXTREME WEIGHT LOSS HYPNOSIS FOR WOMEN

Table Of Contents

GASTRIC BAND HYPNOSIS EXTREME WEIGHT LOSS

Table Of Contents

EXTREME WEIGHT LOSS HYPNOSIS FOR WOMEN

Reprogram Your Subconscious to Lose Weight Without Effort Control Your Mind And Change Your Food Habits Stop Emotional Eating And Increase Your Wellbeing

Introduction

O besity is rising rapidly in the world and is becoming one of the most significant problems for the urban population. Individuals do all kinds of things, mainly physical workouts, to lose weight, but only a small portion takes nutritious foods into account. Over time most people are used to these patterns, which makes the fight much harder to lose weight. Here weight loss with hypnosis is beneficial, but conclusive findings have not been confirmed scientifically.

First of all, weight loss by hypnosis is not immediate but happens after a person has changed his / her ideas and habits. Therefore, a person begins to lose weight. Hypnotherapists mix images, thoughts, and words and bring them to the mind of a person in order to change the body's picture, perception, and belief. A person is thus prepared to adopt healthy habits to lose weight. Hypnosis can only be used to lose weight if this is done together with other strategies, such as exercise.

It is important to note that it is not for everybody to lose weight using the hypnosis process. To be open to this process, you must be prepared to be hypnotized. Secondly, you need to have complete faith in the hypnotherapist and the techniques used. If you are unable to submit your mind to the guidance of hypnotherapists, it may be a waste of time to undertake the procedure. Besides hypnosis, binaural and isochoric beats may be used to help them lose weight. These beats help reprogram the subconscious mind with frequencies of 4-8 Hz that activate the Theta state of mind.

This state corresponds to a profound trance and is easily achieved by skilled mediators. Monaural beats are also instrumental in weight loss, but most people say isochoric tones are much more useful. Such types of brainwave training mainly influence a person's general health over their weight to alter his or her mind. By changing the emphasis from weight loss to wellbeing, the approach begins to change one to a better mental status that benefits from the fact that it attracts the like. If a person concentrates on the negative aspects of weight loss, he attracts more people than he needs.

Hypnosis, also known as hypnotherapy, refers to the profoundly relaxed, almost transitory state of people. However, people are far more open to suggestions in this society.

When an individual is hypnotized, he also is exceptionally calm. You can focus more quickly than "wake up" and consider constructive ideas that enter the subconscious mind. Such suggestions are useful if the person is awake. A reliable therapist takes the patient time. They're going to communicate with them. And the therapist can try to communicate with the client in the subconscious while the client becomes hypnotized. The psychiatrist would be just like an investigator who tries to find the underlying factor that triggers abuse or unethical behavior.

Using binaural beats, which have been clinically proved to work for everyone, one should concentrate on positive aspects of body health. As a result, you gain better health and ultimately meet other healthier bodies. The use of binaural weight loss beats is much simpler and faster than different approaches, such as food plans and weight loss pills. Of course, other things do need to be done to do so, but binaural beats make the procedure much simpler and more pleasant compared to weight loss in hypnosis.

Weight Loss Through Hypnosis

Hypnosis is a method that is to make suggestions to the hypnotized person placed into an altered state of mind with the intention of ringing in the positive changes in their thought and behavior. If the hypnotized person regains consciousness, he or she may continue to act on your subconscious mind's suggestions while hypnotized.

This is standard practice for a therapist to communicate with the subconscious mind of the patient to attempt to determine the underlying factors behind the patient's abuse. When you have trouble maintaining optimal body weight, try using hypnosis weight loss. In the conscious state, which has challenging time security from overeating, you'll try, but in his attempt to lose weight, he'll soon overcome the best intentions and fail.

In such cases, you must seriously consider weight loss by hypnosis and be able to fight at will without your conscious mind rejecting their efforts. Everything that means losing weight by hypnosis is pushing optimistic thoughts into the subconscious mind instead of doing it consciously. Weight reduction by surgery has a higher chance of success as they change their work culture from the inside out, and reprogramming the subconscious mind will change things for the better, with less brain-conscious resistance.

Using weight loss by hypnosis, you can find that after a diet once appeared challenging to maintain, and the explanation for this change for the better is that the relationship with food has undergone a dramatic shift—without ever knowing its—consciously.

We soon realize that weight loss by hypnosis has made it possible to lead a healthier life and will not find it challenging to make the right choices about a balanced diet. Yeah, he'll also get great pleasure and happiness from his new thinking. Moreover, when the brain sends signals to rescheduling the body's commands, you can even notice changes (positive) happening at the cellular level.

Weight-control hypnosis had also worked when other, more traditional weight-loss methods failed. It can also gain a benefit when coping with weight loss by hypnosis as destroying the cravings to overeat, feeling a strong sense of self-empowerment, improving self-esteem, giving you a more positive image, reducing stress levels, and finally finding out what caused you to overeat first.

Myth and Fact of Weight Loss Through Hypnosis

Hypnosis weight loss, is that a fact? Is that all a bunch of lies? Will people really believe that you can actually extract fat from your body through a method that is as controversial as hypnosis? Okay, believe it or not, many studies have shown the efficacy and truthfulness of this technique and, while weight loss due to hypnosis does not work for everyone in the world, it certainly worth your time because it has been beneficial for thousands of people.

You see, all the temperament is hypnosis. If you can change someone's ability to do it (or avoid doing it in this respect), can you finally change their way of living? That's a reality, and hypnosis means that you can alter how someone behaves or even thinks. And here's where hypnosis weight loss comes into play; actually, it's not that hard to change people's thoughts into healthier people, and hypnosis is based directly on people's subconsciousness; programming their weight loss behavior is natural.

However, this method only works for people willing to be hypnotized. There are plenty of people out there for whom hypnosis is entirely ineffective, primarily due to their thought and impermeability to their values and beliefs. If you're such a person, then weight loss by hypnosis would be an excellent failure, but if you're open to new ideas and strategies, your mind may be sensitive to anesthesia, and you could start losing enormous amounts of weight after hypnotizing.

Bear in mind that weight loss by hypnosis extends to several different places to tackle the issue; it's not because you're going to lose this weight miraculously; it means you're going actually to want to pursue a weight loss program and that your willpower will be significantly improved, helping you to stick on the weight loss path without feeling the temptation to drop out.

It is also important to remember that if you want to pursue weight loss through the hypnosis system, you consider all the implications this might have. You must invite an outsider into the depths of your mind and give him permission to reprogram the very principles of life you have created in your life. This doesn't necessarily mean something negative, but it's essential to take note of that before you attempt to sign up for a weight loss by hypnosis program.

CHAPTER 1:

What Hypnosis Is

Throughout our lives, the human brain works continuously. It works instinctively for other behaviors, including breathing: we need not worry about breathing. Hypnosis allows and abuses this unconscious side. Occasionally, hypnosis denials differ from therapist to therapist.

How to define hypnosis? The concept of hypnosis officially refers to an "adjusted state of consciousness," a condition that can be caused by a specialist but also by ourselves. Often, during the watching of a film, the hypnotic state is routinely entered a time of great focus or, on the contrary, when one "picks up" from reality and one starts to daydream. The mind is then either concentrated on a thought or released completely and allows itself to go into its imagination. In these two cases, we are spared by the definition of time. Many examples of the altered state of consciousness are sleep, trance, or even vision.

There are different modalities of hypnosis. The trance occurs naturally and spontaneously, achieving learning and openness of mind. Instead, classical hypnosis is based on the state of loss of consciousness, through receiving direct suggestions from the therapist, through a formal ritual, for trance to occur. Its purpose is to eliminate the symptom.

Ericksonian hypnosis aims to create new experiences that allow us to have a different point of the symptom, understand it better, and replace it with more adaptive behavior.

In the same way that cognitive therapies, one of the objectives of Ericksonian hypnosis is the reorganization of the cognitive structures of the person who attends therapy. Hypnosis encourages her to carry out this process of restructuring without rational and conscious control so that structures inaccessible to consciousness can be modified.

Hypnosis is based on the connection with the unconscious, leaving critical thinking in the background in order to access the person's own resources, resources that, on the other hand, maybe unknown to the person himself. This allows you to get to know yourself better, reduce symptoms, and react more adaptively.

Hypnosis and Relaxation

Normally the process of hypnosis involves the relaxation of the patient, but the relaxation is not necessary for hypnosis nor the fact close your eyes. There is also awake hypnosis, which can be done with the eyes open. Therefore, relaxation is not the same as hypnosis, although it may be helpful. According to Dr. Heap, the most relevant aspect that defines hypnosis is suggestion and suggestibility.

Generally, a hypnosis session begins with a "hypnotic induction." It consists of a series of suggestions that aim to help the person focus on his own sensory experience. The therapist does not express orders or give direct instructions that are difficult to oppose. This could create more resistance and achieve the opposite effect; that is, the person does not want to visualize or do what they propose. In some way, hypnosis could be understood as self-hypnosis.

The psychologist proposes, but it is the person himself who really ends up choosing whether or not to access the suggestions.

There are several factors that influence the degree of suggestibility:

- The person, with his expectations, beliefs, motivation, imaginative capacity, etc

- The therapist, with his communicative style, hypnotic procedures, and patient resistance management, among others

- The therapeutic relationship; is the bond and trust between the therapist and the patient.

During hypnosis, the experiences can seem very real and intense (especially when there is a high degree of suggestibility). It is as if a movie is being watched. You pay attention to what is being watched, and it can be processed as if it were real. This process is possible, thanks to the suggestion.

Talking About Manipulation

Due to the influence of the media, such as movies and television shows, hypnosis has sometimes been associated and is associated with psychological manipulation, although in reality, they have very little to do with it. The only characteristic that relates to them is the increased suggestibility that occurs both in hypnotic processes and in manipulations.

The main difference is that during hypnosis, the person can easily get out of this state of increased suggestibility, while in abusive and manipulative contexts, the return can be hindered. Therefore, it is not manipulation since it cannot induce the person to do something against his will. Furthermore, it retains the ability to interrupt the hypnotic process if desired.

Major Benefits of Hypnosis

Hypnosis is known as a state of mind in which another person induces him to do what is suggested. This is a proven technique, which can be performed either by a hypnotist or by the subject itself. There are many forms of hypnosis, but classical hypnosis, Ericksonian and NLP hypnosis are the three main ones. In certain ways, these three forms of hypnosis can be different, but all have the same aim-to offer an individual benefit.

Hypnosis can be a valuable resource for helping us all-cure illness, relieve stress, and avoid health issues. Nonetheless, hypnosis has major benefits that people need to know and get hold of. The following are some of the big advantages that hypnosis brings:

- **Hypnosis can be used for stress management:** Hypnosis will help your body relax and free your mind from trouble and horrendous thinking. This form of treatment can be performed by a hypnotist, or the individual himself can do it—which is called self-hypnosis. The advice given to the patient by a hypnotist will help him alleviate anxiety, boost mood, feel more confident and relaxed. On the other hand, self-hypnosis can be performed and practiced in a lot of ways—just to make sure a true expert like Igor Ledochowski knows about it.

- **Hypnosis can help a person quit smoking:** Studies show that hypnosis will gradually help a person get rid of their smoking habits and finally quit. Via hypnosis, an individual is more likely to follow the hypnotist's suggestions and do so. Although it works for others, it may not work for others because it also typically depends on several factors, including the particular characteristics of an individual.

- **Hypnosis is a powerful tool in losing weight:** Hypnosis can help a person lose weight as the advice they receive will have a significant impact on creating new healthier behaviors for them to pursue in their altered state of mind. Such healthy habits can help them think positively about weight loss and a healthy lifestyle.

- **It can help treat asthma and phobias:** Hypnosis can be effective in treating phobias almost the same as helping a person quit smoking, as people in this state of mind are more receptive to advice and can take the guidance offered by hypnotists positively.

The reason phobias exist in the unconscious part of our minds is why Hypnotherapy and NLP are so effective in the treatment of phobias. Indeed, if you suffer from a phobia, you are possibly aware of its irrational existence but yet unable to resolve it with your conscious mind. Several studies also indicate that hypnosis can help improve children's asthma symptoms, but this is still early to conclude.

The Power of Hypnosis

There are many benefits of conversational hypnosis, as the power of hypnosis will allow you to do many things you never dreamed of. A course on hypnosis will make you manipulate everyone to follow your lead, get clients and customers to eat from your mouth, order respect, negotiate effectively, hold loyal lovers 24/7, and make everyone consent to your point of view, including obedience from teens and kids.

There are ways to do it unconventionally, and if you know how to do hypnosis, you should do it. Everyone has the potential to hypnotize because it is normal among men and women, and they can do it easily if they complete a course on the subject rather than fishing in the dark. Using conversational hypnosis, as described by the name on the website, you can actually do things that others cannot conceive of.

By learning how to hypnotize somebody, you might be on the way to manipulating that specific person's power of hypnosis and make him or her follow the orders. How to do a hypnosis guide will help you launch the exploration to read every customer of yours like an open book. Only flit through the person's mind, and the entire person will be exposed to you like a journal.

You can understand and know the mind because you can learn how to interpret someone else's mind. With a single command, you can make them change their attitudes and, with a series of commands, you can gradually gain power over the individual and fine-tuning responses to your wishes. You'll know what he or she is thinking and how to turn a "no" with a few commands into a "yes."

Hypnosis could allow you to do amazing things. You can easily train people to respond to your voice tones the way you want and continually bid. You will know that you can fine-tune thoughts to strengthen relationships and build the missing bond between people. It's not a spell, but a course that's science, helping many people from coast to coast.

During daily interactions, you can use hypnosis because communication is the way to manipulate people and make them offer. This will not only help you excel in your career but also help you load your day-to-day activities. Earlier, physicians were barred from hypnosis, but later, the rule changed and saved lives. You, too, will practice conversational hypnosis if you want to practice hypnosis and unlock the strength of your hypnosis.

The Power of Hypnosis for Weight Loss

Many people will try anything when it comes to weight loss—anything to stop normal diet and exercise. One of the more unorthodox approaches you do not find is weight loss hypnosis. Many hypnosis weight loss services claim to be able to get rid of old habits, including eating too much fast food. Hypnosis works by putting you in a deep sleep where your mind is open to suggestions. For example, the hypnotist will convince you that you no longer have cravings or anything similar.

Some people believe that hypnosis is a crock, while others swear. Specific outcomes can differ—if you were hypnotized successfully before. This form of hypnosis will work for you. When contemplating weight loss hypnosis, realism is critical. Hypnosis won't make you shed pounds overnight. Perhaps it will disappear your cravings or make you want more exercise. The results will be sluggish.

One thing to stop when searching for weight loss hypnosis is hypnosis services in audiotape format. These programs say you can easily get rid of your poor eating and exercise habits by listening to a tape repeatedly. If the whole thing sounds crazy to you, well, you're right. If you're seriously contemplating weight loss hypnosis, you can see a licensed clinical hypnotist and see whether it will work.

CHAPTER 5:

How Hypnosis Works for Weight Loss

Until dealing with whether or not hypnosis works for weight loss, it is important to consider hypnosis as a whole subject or technique. Hypnosis is characterized as a trance-like mental state induced by enticing techniques and methodologies, typically a verbal guidance method and beginning with relaxation suggestions. A hypnotist can cause hypnosis, or sometimes even self-induced.

How does hypnosis contribute to weight loss? Hypnosis is something we usually see as entertainment, but have you ever considered weight loss hypnosis? Trying to use hypnosis to cope with an issue as extreme as obesity is easy to be cynical, but maybe it's not as crazy as it sounds. Hypnosis for weight loss is definitely an interesting concept - it offers people a fairly simple way out of their weight issue by avoiding food cravings at the source.

One weight-loss problem with hypnosis is the same problem that plagues most weight-loss remedies. There's plenty of scams out there, and those behind them won't think twice about trying to steal your money for a product that doesn't do anything. Hypnosis has the same problem. You may be able to trust certain statements about weight loss therapy for hypnosis, but many of them are full of lies.

In such cases, the old adage typically holds true: if anything seems too good to be true, it probably is. When hypnosis for weight loss treatment promises to help you shed some insane weight in few weeks or similar exaggerations, it's pretty safe to say it's a scam. If you find reports claiming that hypnosis can fully alter the way the mind works to avoid feeding, they're probably false.

The truth remains that hypnosis will help you lose weight. It's just that it won't make love handles melt away overnight. Hypnosis is more science than magic-all; it is when a person enters a state of intense, relaxed focus where they become more suggestive. This means thoughts put into a person's head during a session of hypnosis are much more likely to stick.

A hypnosis session won't turn you into a robot that's immune to cravings and programmed not to over-eat. What it can do is make a person more likely to adopt a proper dietary plan. The effects are solely emotional. Hypnosis can't "convince" your body to promote weight loss, and it can just implant the idea in your brain that you don't need to eat the second piece of cake.

Individuals pursuing hypnotic weight-loss approaches should be especially cautious about group hypnosis sessions. To properly function, hypnosis must be personalized specifically to the person receiving it. Community sessions obviously won't work because the hypnotist can't communicate with someone on his own. You should be cautioned against hypnosis cassettes or videos, as they share the same problem.

The hypnosis of weight loss is very enticing. If you can train your mind to reduce your cravings and improve your willpower, you're on your way to weight loss. Be vigilant and research all the choices before you purchase a drug or see a hypnotist, or else you may end up with nothing at all.

Every overweight person in the world seeks weight loss techniques. Many people are also willing to do something to make those extra kilos look appealing. The weight loss industry is making millions of dollars, and people cannot achieve what they want.

Recently, studies have shown that hypnosis can assist in weight loss. However, hypnosis is not a treatment that can help a person lose extra weight overnight. Weight loss hypnosis is a method used to concentrate people on their goals. It should be remembered that many people with disabilities and addiction issues were able to overcome their problems through hypnosis, and the same concepts apply to weight loss.

For a weight loss hypnosis program, a hypnotherapist first recognizes the goals a person needs to accomplish and analyze the actual state of the person. You would also find eating habits and other factors that keep it from losing weight. Based on these findings, he will develop a system and reflect on his suggestions while in the hypnotic state.

It can take quite a number of visits to produce results. The hypnotherapist can plant positive advice and ideas in the minds of the individual trying to lose weight. Hearing the same points and suggestions would improve his commitment and determination and make him do everything possible to lose weight and therefore stop all obstacles that hinder him from achieving his target.

Hypnosis for Weight Loss ant the Way It Works

Diet, exercise, and weight loss are maybe some of the most hated things that most people have to do in life, and some of their most difficult things. When you are out of shape, it is a daunting struggle to get back into form. Weight loss hypnosis is one method that people are constantly using to try and get back into healthier lifestyles. This sounds like a brilliant idea for many people, but they don't really know how anything like this works. This is a short description of how weight loss hypnosis is working.

The goal is to alter how the subconscious works, like all the hypnosis plans. Training your subconscious will change your thoughts and actions and will catapult you toward meaningful changes in your life. I assume most people know hypnosis to avoid unhealthy habits such as alcohol and smoking. Through changing the subconscious, your appetite, and your need for these things, you can regulate your pressures. For weight loss hypnosis, the same basic concepts are employed.

The purpose of the hypnosis of weight loss is to improve yourself over time; this is not an instant cure that can shed pounds within the first week. Rather, you stop eating fast food over time because it doesn't taste nearly as good, stop buying pizzas, stop eating when you are nervous or excited. After all, stop eating out of the habit. It is a tool to encourage you to turn to healthy eating by substituting good food for bad foods.

You learn how to eat well, and how to spend 20 minutes walking during your lunch break can improve your life's health. It won't instantly lose weight or change your life. It is possible to do this hypnosis in several different ways, including qualified individuals, DVDs, and even self-hypnosis. You will have to study the choice between these different choices to determine what is right for you individually.

In modern days, weight is a constant problem, everybody tries to get in shape, they try, but success lags behind. There are so many items that treat the body. When you try like most people, something is lacking in a weight-loss equation, you can try the sequence of "tested" diets and the most amazing exercises to get in shape, but if you don't care about giving the extra help to weight loss, the fight is already lost, it doesn't take long before you regain it. The answer is to train the mind, and weight loss hypnosis is the best thing.

It helps you find new opportunities for achieving your target by using hypnosis for weight loss. Experts say there are four effective ways to achieve your goal. The first approach is to imagine the dream body with your inner eyes, how it feels, and how you walk around. Repeat these pictures every day, and your plans will be much easier to execute. The second approach is to listen to subliminal messages that are intended as weight loss hypnosis. Listen to the tape or CD before going to bed. This works the following way, transmitting messages to the extremely sensitive subconscious mind. You will note any improvements when you wake up, and do not forget to repeat the cycle every night.

Another effective hypnosis for weight loss is to overcome the stress problems; some studies indicate that people have great trouble losing weight if they cannot cope effectively with stress every day. The first step is to identify the key causes of stress and solve them by relaxation when coping with these issues and then concentrate on the weight problem.

And the final approach is by thinking positive motivational thoughts by using weight loss hypnosis. There is a basic universe rule that does what we want; the more we want it to be, the more easily it is real, be it good or bad. The rational approach is, therefore, not to use positive thought, so hypnosis for weight loss is a good idea for you.

Mastering the Magic of Hypnosis of Weight Loss

Hypnosis for weight loss has now become much more common. After the discovery, the brain plays a significant role in weight loss. It actually plays a greater role than most people expect or assume. People who haven't been on a weight loss plan will not understand this easily.

It is also said that the human fault is overweight. You may also have learned that you will stop eating and start exercising to lose weight. Most people who struggle with weight loss have done many things to lose their weight but have obtained little to no positive results.

Although it is important to recognize certain factors that are responsible for weight gain and likely clarify the reasons why tentative weight loss attempts have failed, it does not go beyond this. Some claim that acquiring information and awareness about the cause of weight loss and why efforts to lose weight failed is part of the fight for weight loss.

If you know this is half the fight for weight loss, you can definitely be considered the easiest part. Someone who wants to lose weight is already aware of what holds them off. What they don't know is how they would fix this.

Talk therapy has become very common these days, allowing people to change their minds and regulate their body weight better. There are various forms of speech therapy, but weight loss hypnosis has taken center stage. While hypnosis can sound like an older term, it is one of the treatment methods frequently used by healthcare professionals and clinics for weight loss as it has proven to be highly successful in most patients.

The weight loss hypnosis is prescribed and favored due to the fast results that are long-term, like in computer therapy or psychoanalysis. Hypnosis is a special technique, as it focuses primarily on positive factors that have changed the patient's body and mind.

Although most psychoanalytical approaches seek to explore the causes behind weight loss issues, hypnosis easily works through and removes those barriers and thus provides an early road to weight loss. Hypnosis may simply be described as the ability to rewrite unconsciously and consciously the actions and the thoughts that go through your mind.

Weight loss hypnosis uses relaxation and repetition. The sessions typically consist of 20 to 30 minutes of guided and repeated meditation every day. When administered for a continuous 30-day duration, the brain adopts a new style of thought or behaviors.

For most instances, the human brain consumes all that it experiences or sees through layers of consciousness. When a person hears or sees something, it is stored in the short memory of the brain. The data accumulated in the short memory will serve as a permanent influence on the mind, contributing to new patterns or beliefs.

CHAPTER 6:

Self-Hypnosis for Weight Loss

O ne of the hardest parts about losing weight is having to wait so long to see the results. While there isn't a way to lose 20 pounds overnight, you can reshape your mentality to grow your patience for the process. When you fully recognize the time and how that plays into weight loss, you won't be looking at the scale every hour, begging for results. Instead, you will be happy with your journey and recognize the incredible way your body is changing. This is a visualization exercise that will help you get in the right mindset to lose weight fast.

We all want time just to relax, dream, pretend. It refreshes the physical body and rejuvenates the spirit. It gives us just that when we practice our hypnosis: a very personal moment to animate and be able to enrich our mind and body. The procedure is over. You need nothing more than a secure and comfortable venue.

Performing for Self-Hypnosis

There are certain guidelines for hypnosis, and they make sure the practice is the most effective and has the greatest advantages. Find a convenient and quiet spot in your home or office when you're ready to start using the audio, where you can sit in a chair, recline, or even lie down. Make sure you're comfortable, and you don't have to pay attention to anything else in a spot. Do not listen to your work on trance while driving a car or running any kind of machinery. To properly practice your self-hypnosis, it is helpful to agree on a daily time each day or night. Bedtime is a perfect opportunity to enjoy your job in a trance, and training at this time can be a wonderful way to reach a restful sleep.

Distractions and interruptions are possible. You are using them instead of making them torment you and drive you away from your job in a trance. To enhance your experience of trance, use the sounds in the environment around you. For example, you might hear a sound while doing your hypnosis and start thinking that it distracts you. You then concentrate more on the diversion than on your hypnosis. You may be tempted to fight it—which takes energy off the hypnosis. Instead, when you notice a sound that appears distracting or annoying at first, take control of it by giving it your permission as a background sound to be here. Distractions also include the feelings you can feel in yourself. You may find yourself feeling, for example, a part of your body that itches. The more you focus on itching or scratching the itch, the less you concentrate on the trance. You are just reminding yourself at those times that you have permission to move your attention back to your trance or daydream and let the itch unravel. We teach patients a similar way of focusing attention away from the "distraction" of pain when working with them. We can't control the world around us or the sensations within us, after all, but we can choose where to focus our attention. If you have trouble letting go of an annoying distraction, you may need to order it as a background sound or feeling, allowing you to go inside more comfortably. Detach yourself from anything your commitment to your hypnosis is competing with. Let go of any dispute with the world. Just let it be there, and you won't notice it again sooner or later. Once you learn to accept a feeling, a noise, or other factors that interfere with your hypnosis, you don't let it affect you longer.

Step-by-Step Guide in Self-hypnotization

This meditation is going to be a visualization. You will want to make sure that you are in a comfortable place where you can drift off and go to sleep if you want to. We will take you through the scene that will await you at the end of your natural weight loss journey. Close your eyes, and keep your body as relaxed as possible. Start to focus on your breathing. Breathe in through your nose and out through your mouth. Concentrate the air as it travels through your body so that you will be able to shut out any negative or toxic thoughts more easily than you have at this moment.

Focus on your breathing and breathe in for five and out for five. We are going to count down through 10 a few times to get you in the right mindset.

- Breathe in now for the count from 1-10

- Now we are going to count down from 10. Make sure that you are still focused on breathing in this pattern.

- Count down from 10.

- You see nothing around you. Everything is black, and you are completely relaxed.

You are completely quiet and serene. Your body is feeling free and relaxed. You look ahead of you, and you start to see a little white dot. This white dot continues to grow and grow and grow until it has engulfed you.

You see a clear blue sky with the sun shining down. The white comes from the bright gravel driveway that's in front of you. You start to walk towards a gigantic mansion. You take a few steps up and notice the marble front doors in front of you. You are looking out, and you see nothing but a green grassy pasture and skyline dotted with trees. You are completely centered and peaceful at this moment. You reach your hand out and grasp the brass knob right in front of you.

Your body is pure and healthy. You don't have any marks from surgeries or the sign of starvation in your eyes. You are happy because you have completed this task naturally. You worked alongside your body to get the results that you not only want but also deserve. You look around you and see that you have managed to create this life. You have your dream body with your dream hair and a happy shining face, and you are surrounded by everything you could ever want. You notice there's a long hallway, and you hear some chatter at the end. Before following, you stop first into a bedroom against a long hallway. On the bed, you see a gorgeous outfit you could ever imagine. It has all the makings of something that helps you to look good and makes you feel good. You slip into this outfit now and take a look in the mirror. Once again, your incredibly defined body shows through this silhouette. You exude confidence. It doesn't even matter what you're wearing, but this outfit, in particular, makes you feel like a luxury.

You start to admire your body from the bottom up. You notice your incredible feet and how they have been able to carry you throughout this whole process. You have shoes that comfortably fit, and your body is no longer sore. You can easily move your ankles and your feet around as needed. They carry you to places that you never thought you would find yourself. They have been able to hold your entire body. Without these powerful feet, you would not have been able to go through this whole process. You move on up now to your calves. You see, these intense calves combine with your shins, and understand how they have also helped to push you forward. You were able to run and walk on these calves to burn so many calories. You naturally used this small part of your body to have so much powerful force. You were able to lift weights, and you were able to do squats, jumping jacks, and other fun exercises. They help you dance. Each time you move your calf, you notice that this is something so powerful and strong. That helped you through this journey. Moving up, you see your knees and your thighs. This part helped you bend, and you were able to stretch and feel your muscles relax as you worked them out.

You're able to recognize all of the powerful and incredible ways that your legs have carried you throughout this life. They have helped you run, exercise, and jog, along with other physical exercise methods, so that you can get the body that you desire. These incredible legs look so great in the mirror as you look in front of you. You are not afraid to show them off anymore. They are a part of who you are. You see your stomach now, and it shows just how incredibly strong your willpower is. You've been able to say no to food that you know not only adds extra weight to your body but just generally makes you feel bad.

You don't have that big gut anymore that is filled with foods that are unhealthy. Having a belly is not bad at all. Most animals even need this belly. However, your gut isn't one that weighs you down. You don't feel so full and greasy in your stomach. You feel good. You know that you've been working with your gut healthily and happily to provide it with everything you need. You haven't been feeding it food that makes it feel bad. You only give it good nutritious food that is easy for it to process. It breaks down your food and takes every mineral, vitamin, and nutrient from this substance to make you feel better. Your stomach knows what to do with food exactly and where to send the various parts that it breaks down.

There is nothing that is going to kill your confidence. Now, you might still have certain goals for your body and want to lose more weight, but overall, you feel incredible. You've seen your future, and it is bright.

You take a step in, and everybody simply gives you a handshake or a pat on the back. They smile and lift their drinks to you, acknowledging all of the hard work that you put in. Everybody knows that this isn't something simple. You can see on their faces that they might even want it themselves, but they didn't have the strong willpower that you had. You were able to create this incredible life for yourself. You've managed to get everything that you could have ever wanted. No longer is it a fantasy. This is what is needed exactly for your confidence. You are filled with joy. Now that you've seen this visualization, you understand that you can see the future. This weight loss journey is going to happen so quickly. Before you know it, you will be the one walking through this mansion. Notice your breathing once again.

Breathe in for count down from 10.

We are going to count down once more, and as we do, you're either going to drift off to sleep or move on to another meditation. You know what you exactly have to do to get the quick and easy natural weight loss results that you want for a better life. Don't forget your castle and the reality that awaits you.

Count down from 20.

CHAPTER 7:

The Power of Hypnosis and Self-Hypnosis and How to Use Them Successfully

Self-hypnosis has a powerful ability to help you accomplish virtually anything you desire to achieve. Whether you want to reduce or manage stress, motivate yourself to achieve something, relax from stress or other upsetting emotions, concentrate more efficiently or effectively on a task at hand, or direct yourself to do or accomplish something, self-hypnosis can help you drastically.

How to Enter a Hypnotic State

When it comes to effectively making use of self-hypnosis, it is generally important that a person has first experienced hypnosis in some other form. This can include attending a professional hypnotherapist and being hypnotized, or it may include regular practice through guided hypnosis sessions that may be retrieved through audio files. An individual first must learn to become familiar with the hypnotic state and what it feels like before embarking on self-hypnosis, as this will ensure that they are clear on what to look for and what to expect. While you can certainly engage in self-hypnosis without prior experience or practice, this may reduce results and benefits as you may not be clear on what to expect or how the experience or process should be facilitated.

Once you have already experienced some form of hypnosis, you should have a fairly good idea of what to expect and what will be experienced during the process. You will be familiar with how the hypnotic state is achieved, what it feels like, and what happens once you have entered a hypnotic state. From there, you can follow these same practices to achieve the hypnotic state in your self-hypnosis practice.

The hypnotic state is not guided by an external influence when it comes to self-hypnosis. Instead, it is achieved through facilitating deep relaxation within yourself and your body. You do this through a series of breathing practices and intentions, whereby you clear your mind and focus solely on your body and breath. This is very similar to meditation practice, so people who are already fluent in achieving a relaxed state through meditation will have a general idea of how self-hypnosis can be achieved. If you have not practiced meditation in the past, it may be ideal to begin your practice now so that you can practice entering a deep state of relaxation that allows your mind to be influenced by hypnosis.

How to Be Guided

When it comes to self-hypnosis, you are guided by yourself. This comes through self-suggestion, as well as self-exploration. The best way to guide yourself through an intentional hypnosis practice is to set the expectation of what you want to be guided through or toward before you enter the hypnotic state. For example, say that you want to hypnotize yourself and practice self-hypnosis as a means to help you quit something, such as smoking. Before entering the state of deep relaxation that is required for hypnosis, you would set this intention and repeat it to yourself over and over again. Then, you would begin working on setting yourself into the hypnotic state of deep relaxation. Once you are in that state, you can begin repeating the intention over and over once again. This will set the intention into your mind and allow the message to sink even deeper into your subconscious, allowing it to help rewrite and reprogram your subconscious just as any other form or state of hypnosis would.

Being in a state of both physical and mental deep relaxation such as that which is experienced when you are undergoing hypnosis means that the intention you set and the message you repeat goes far beyond your conscious mind. Your conscious mind is the "first step" of your mind that is used to process information. This part of your mind will easily attest or contest anything that you feed your mind with. The idea is that you allow yourself to enter a deep state of relaxation and then begin directing your mind through intention, which results in these intentions bypassing your conscious mind and entering your subconscious or unconscious mind, which is the one that is responsible for all that you do. This results in information that may no longer be serving you being redesigned by your intention, making it easier for you to facilitate complete changes.

Achieve Results Through This

The ability to achieve results through self-hypnosis works the same as your ability to achieve results through any form of hypnosis. Whether we realize it or not, our subconscious or unconscious mind is directly responsible for virtually everything that we do. This is where our "survival" information is stored. Anything that urges us to jump into action or produce certain results are all stored within this part of our mind and is responsible for virtually everything that we do. From breathing and digesting food that we eat to telling us who to trust and who not to, and even helping us make an opinion about things and form judgments on various topics, our subconscious mind is directly responsible for these actions.

The conscious mind can recognize and become aware of things, but it is not directly responsible for what we ultimately choose to do. So, by consciously choosing to make a change, we must then relay that change into our subconscious so that it happens. Just as with any other form of hypnosis, performing self-hypnosis allows you to take a conscious desire to change and relay it back into your subconscious mind so that it takes effect, and true changes are seen and experienced in our lives. For example, if you want to stop biting your nails, you may tell your conscious mind that you want to do so. Then, later, you begin biting your nails without realizing it because it is a practice that has become a part of your subconscious psyche. Therefore, if you want to instill real change, you have to bypass your conscious mind and directly tell your subconscious mind to change this behavior. This is achieved through self-hypnosis and intention, and the results can be just as powerful as any other form of hypnosis.

The Big Difference

There truly is no significant difference between regular hypnosis and self-hypnosis, aside from who is facilitating the hypnotic state and directing the subconscious mind in that state. As we have already talked about, hypnosis is something that is facilitated by a third-party to direct the relationship between your conscious and unconscious mind. Self-hypnosis, however, is done directly between your conscious and unconscious mind and allows you to perform the practice at any given time, in any given place, for any particular reason.

Choosing between self-hypnosis and hypnosis is personal, and both have their unique benefits that outweigh the benefits given by the other. For example, if you are inexperienced and are looking to be hypnotized by a professional to achieve something big, such as to motivate yourself to lose weight or become healthier, professional hypnosis can help you facilitate this change. Professional hypnosis will be able to facilitate quicker results than an inexperienced self-hypnosis practitioner, and they will also be able to use a broader range of words and intentions because they are not in the hypnotic state, but rather you are, and they are simply directing it. By this understanding, a hypnotherapist can take you through a broader range of intentions and experiences when it comes to hypnosis.

However, professional hypnotherapists can become rather costly and may not always be able to provide you with the level of help that you need for various intentions. For example, they may not entirely understand what change you want to make, they may not be within your budget, or they may simply not be available at the exact times that you need hypnosis to help you. In these cases, self-hypnosis is a great option. You can enter a hypnotic state and then focus on your intention and, as a result, facilitate change directly at the moment that change is needed. This can increase the benefits and results you experience from your hypnosis, and it can make hypnotherapy more effective for you.

If you are wondering which to choose: hypnosis with a professional hypnotherapist or self-hypnosis, the best answer is likely to choose both. Seeking help from a professional hypnotherapist can help you learn about hypnosis and begin navigating the world of hypnotherapy and facilitate major changes in a shorter amount of time. Then, coupling this practice with a self-hypnosis practice can help you get the most out of your experience and see greater results. You can engage in shorter, more direct self-hypnotherapy sessions as needed to supplement your professional hypnotherapist's results and ultimately facilitate a total change.

As you become more practiced with self-hypnosis, you may begin to discover that you no longer need as much help from professional hypnotherapists. While seeking professional help in the face of major, difficult, or stubborn changes may be desirable, you will likely find that you can facilitate major changes in a shorter time, the more you practice. For that reason, you become your change-maker and influencer. This can make the idea of increasing your skills around self-hypnosis more desirable and can prove why it is important to begin practicing and taking advantage of this incredible practice as soon as possible.

CHAPTER 8:

Hypnosis Method

If you can afford to undergo a series of hypnotherapy sessions with a specialist, you may do so. This is ideal as you will work with a professional who can guide you through the treatment and will also provide you with valuable advice on nutrition and exercises.

Clinical Hypnotherapy

During your first session, your therapist will usually start by explaining to you the type of hypnotherapy he or she is using. Then you will discuss your personal goals so the therapist can understand your motivations better.

The formal session will start with your therapist, speaking in a gentle and soothing voice. This will help you relax and feel safe during the entire therapy. Once your mind is more receptive, the therapist will start suggesting ways that can help you modify your exercise or eating habits as well as other ways to help you reach your weight loss goals.

Specific words or repetition of specific phrases can help you at this stage. The therapist may also help you in visualizing the body image you want, which is one effective technique in hypnotherapy.

To end the session, the therapist will bring you out from the hypnotic stage, and you will start to be more alert. Your personal goals will influence the duration of the hypnotherapy sessions as well as the number of total sessions that you may need. Most people begin to see results in as few as two to four sessions.

DIY Hypnotherapy

If you are not comfortable working with a professional hypnotherapist or you just can't afford the sessions, you can choose to perform self-hypnosis. While this is not as effective as the sessions under a professional, you can still try it and see if it can help you with your weight loss goals.

Here are the steps if you wish to practice self-hypnosis:

- **Believe in the power of hypnotism.** Remember, this alternative treatment requires the person to be open and willing. It will not work for you if your mind is already set against it.

- **Find a comfortable and quiet room to practice hypnotherapy.** Ideally, you should find a room that is free from noise and where no one can disturb you. Wear loose clothes and set relaxing music to help in setting up the mood.

- **Find a focal point.** Choose an object in a room that you can focus on. Use your concentration on this object so you can start clearing your mind of all thoughts.

- **Breathe deeply.** Start with six deep breaths, breathe in through your nose, and breathe out through your mouth.

- **Close your eyes.** Think about your eyelids becoming heavy, and just let them close slowly.

- **Imagine that all stress and tension are coming out of your body.** Let this feeling move down from your head, to your shoulders, to your chest, to your arms, to your stomach, to your legs, and finally to your feet.

- **Clear your mind.** When you are totally relaxed, your mind must be clear, and you can initiate the process of self-hypnotism.

- **Visualize a pendulum**. In your mind, picture a moving pendulum. The movement of the pendulum is popular imagery used in hypnotism to encourage focus.

- **Start visualizing your ideal body image and size.** This should help you instill in your subconscious the importance of a healthy diet and exercise.

- **Suggest to yourself to avoid unhealthy food and start exercising regularly.** You can use a particular mantra such as "I will exercise at least three times a week. Unhealthy food will make me sick."

- **Wake up.** Once you have achieved what you want during hypnosis, you must wake yourself. Start by counting back from one to 10, and wake up when you reach 10.

Remember, a healthy diet doesn't mean that you have to significantly reduce your food intake. Just reduce your intake of food that is not healthy for you. Never hypnotize yourself out of eating. Just suggest to yourself to eat less of the food that you know is just making you fat.

CHAPTER 9:

Portion Control

Whether you wish to shed many pounds or maintain a healthy weight, proper portion consumption is as necessary as the consumption of appropriate foods. The rate of obesity among youngsters and adults has increased partly owing to the increase in restaurant portions.

A portion is the total quantity of food that you eat in one sitting. A serving size is the suggested quantity of one food. For instance, the amount of steak you eat for dinner maybe a portion; however, three ounces of steak, maybe a serving. Controlling serving sizes helps with portion control.

Health Benefits of Portion Control

Serious health problems are caused by overeating—for example, type 2 diabetes, weight problems, high blood pressure, and many more. Therefore, when you are looking to lead a healthy lifestyle, portion control should be a significant priority.

Fullness and Weight Management

Feeling satiable, or having a sense of fullness, will affect the quantity you eat and the way you usually eat. According to the British Nutrition Foundation, slowly eating and smaller portions increase the feeling of satiety after a meal.

Eating smaller parts also permits your body to use the food you eat right away for energy, rather than storing the excess as fat. Losing weight is not as straightforward as solely controlling your portion sizes; however, once you learn to observe the quantity of food you eat, you will begin to apply conscious intake, which might assist you in making healthier food decisions.

When you eat too quickly, you do not notice your stomach's cues that it is full. Eat slowly and listen to hunger cues to enhance feelings of fullness and, ultimately, consume less food.

Improved Digestion

Considerably larger portion sizes contribute to an upset stomach and discomfort (caused by a distended stomach pushing down on your other organs). Your gastrointestinal system functions best when it is not full of food. Managing portions can help to get rid of cramping and bloating after eating. You furthermore may run the danger of getting pyrosis because if you have a full abdomen, it will push hydrochloric acid back into your digestive tract.

Money Savings

Eating smaller parts may lead to monetary benefits, mainly when eating out. In addition to eating controlled serving sizes, you do not have to purchase as many groceries. Dosing the serving proportions can make the cereal box, and the package of nuts last longer than if they are eaten directly from the container.

Adult portion sizes at restaurants will equal two, three, or even more servings. Therefore, immediately after the food arrives at your table, request for a takeaway container and put away half of your food from the plate. Take your food home, and this way, you will have two meals for the worth of one.

How to Control Portions Using Hypnosis

Hypnosis can take you into a deeply relaxed state and quickly train your mind to understand when to do away with excess food instinctively, and allow your digestion to be lighter and more comfortable. You may discover the pleasure of being in tune with what your own body requires for nourishment. Hypnosis will re-educate your instincts to regulate hunger pangs. As you relax and repeatedly listen to powerful hypnotic suggestions that are going to be absorbed by your mind; you may quickly begin to note that:

- Your mind is no longer engrossed in food

- Your abdomen and gut feel lighter

- You now do not feel uncontrollable hunger pangs at "non-meal" times

- You naturally forget to have food between meals

- You begin to enjoy a healthier lifestyle

There is a somewhat simple self-hypnosis process for helping you control your appetite and portions. In a nutshell, you are immersing yourself into a psychological state and picture a dial or a flip switch of some type that is symbolic of your craving and your real hunger. Then you repeatedly apply to develop a true sense of control, then you employ it out of the hypnotic state and when confronted with those things and circumstances to curb the perceived hunger and control your appetite.

Step 1

Get yourself into a comfortable position and one where you will remain undisturbed for the period of this exercise. Make sure your feet are flat on the ground, and your hands are not touching. Then once you are in position, calm yourself.

You can do that by using hypnosis tapes; they are basic processes to assist you in opening the door of your mind.

Step 2

You may prefer to deepen your hypnotic state. The best and most straightforward is imagining yourself in your favorite place and relaxing your body bit by bit. Keep focused on the session at hand (that is, watch out to not drift off), then go to the third step.

Step 3

Take a picture of a dial, a lever, or a flippy switch of some kind that is on a box or mounted on a wall of some sort-let it fully controls your mind's eye. Notice the colors, the materials that it is created out of, and the way it indicates 0-10 to mark the variable degrees of your real hunger.

Notice wherever it is currently indicating; let it show you how hungry you are. Remember when was the last time you ate, what you ate, whether the hunger is genuine or merely reacting to a recent bout of gluttony and wanting to gratify that sensation!

Once you have established the dial, where it is set, and trust that the reading is correct, then go to the subsequent step.

Step 4

Flip the dial down a peg and notice the effects taking place within you. Study your feedback and ascertain that it feels like you are moving your appetite with the dial. The more you believe you are affecting your appetite with the dial, the more practical its application in those real-life situations.

Practice turning it down even lower and start recognizing how you use your mind to change your perceived appetite utilizing a method that is healthy and helps keep you alert when you encounter circumstances with plenty of food supply. Tell yourself that the more you observe this, the better control you gain over your appetite.

You might even create a strong affirmation that accompanies this dial. "I am in control of my eating" is one such straightforward statement. Word it as you wish and make sure it is one thing that resonates well with you. Once you have repeated the meaningful affirmations to yourself severally with conviction, proceed to the following step.

Step 5

Visualize yourself during a future scenario, where there is going to be constant temptation to continue eating although you are full or to consume an excessive amount. See the sights of that place, take a mental note of the other people there, notice the smells, hear the sounds. Become increasingly aware of how you are feeling in this place. Get the most definition and clarity possible, then notice that once the temptation presents itself, you turn down the dial on your craving. You realize that you are not hungry to eat anymore, then repeat the positive affirmations to yourself a few more times to strengthen it.

Run through this future situation severally on loop to make sure your mind is mentally rehearsed about your plan to respond.

Step 6

Twitch your little finger and toes, then open your eyes and proceed to observe your skills in real-life and spot how much control you have.

CHAPTER 10:

Stop Emotional Eating

Most people had eaten at one time or another for emotional reasons. When there's tension, it can be the go-to feeling. I recall several times when one person would say to colleagues, "I'm hungry—who wants to get something with me (meaning something sweet)?" We were all exhausted and knew nothing but eating.

Eating to control emotions can end up having some negative effects over a long period of time. One of the main issues with using food to control emotions is that it can lead to weight problems, and a lot more problems come with weight.

Eating for emotional purposes is used to soothe any of a variety of emotions like depression, rage, disappointment, loneliness, or boredom, to name a few. Emotional hunger isn't the same as physical hunger (the true reason for eating), and you're looking for food to meet emotional needs. We know that food cannot actually fulfill an emotional need, as it is intended to relieve physical hunger.

The starting point for emotional eating is to learn if you're getting involved in it. Verily, many people are unaware of what they are doing, believing that they are actually overeating. Here are some emotional eating signs:

- You eat when you're not hungry

- Eat when you feel like you are

- Eat-in silence

- Eating afterward and feeling guilty

- Eating too much and not knowing why

- Eating to keep yourself feeling better

- For no apparent reason, craving a snack, and feeling you can't live without it.

Emotional eating can be stimulating because, at first, it tastes good, and there are all the optimistic feelings about how much you want or need it. The good feelings (relief, calm) from emotional eating will only last for a certain amount of time (one minute to hours), followed by a turning point where you experience the following situations:

- Appointed guilty

- Feeling humiliated

- Feeling irritated that you are overdoing yourself

- Feeling a revival of the initial sensation causing the binge

- Feel angry that you've lost weight or maybe gained weight

The final end result is that emotional eating doesn't work to relieve the initial emotion that sent you to the food. Understanding this is the starting point for this behavior to shift. Keep it for yourself. Often compliment yourself that you're "getting it" now. You can feel the need to beat yourself to do so for too long. This thinking cycle does not help you in any constructive way, however, but instead bring you back to overeating because you are mad at yourself for overeating (a circular cycle).

How to Stop Emotional Eating

Some of us have participated in emotional eating for some point or another. Emotional eating occurs if we eat to soothe wounded feelings or cope with a stressful situation. Emotional eating can occur after a hard day at work, a fight with a loved one, or when the kids run around the house crying. The first step to avoiding emotional eating is to become conscious that it is occurring. In the course of the day, ask yourself many times how you feel to stop a significant amount of tension. Recognize the symptoms of discomfort or tension. Find a way to convey the feelings efficiently so they can be published. Holding in negative or hurtful feelings may lead to a binge later on. Stopping to evaluate your emotions during the day can also help you pause before reaching for unhealthy foods.

Second, preventing causes. Think back to the last emotional eating moment. What happened just before you'd eat? Remember not being hungry and feeding anyway? Do you still eat after a difficult job meeting or dispute with a co-worker? Identifying and preventing emotional-eating activities can help deter potential occurrences.

Third, try doing something else while eating happens. By monitoring your emotional state during the day, you will be conscious of when emotional eating will occur and seeking solutions to it. When you are eating fattening foods, it makes you feel confident and relaxed, build a list of other habits contributing to the same feelings. Exercise is an important way to promote positive feelings. Other suggestions like hot baths, reading a good book, or watching your favorite movie. Keep the activity list on your refrigerator to remind you of alternative suggestions should a deficiency occur. Journaling is another way to avoid emotional eating.

By tracking feelings all day long, anxieties, fears, and emotions, you will help recognize causes. After keeping a list for a few days, look back for specific feelings that made you eat emotionally, recurring things like job stress that require action to alleviate tension, or situations that make you feel stressed. Another strategy to reduce emotional eating is to cut your portions in half. If you've had a busy day and have a meal, place half-sized portions on your plate and assess how you feel after you've eaten. If you're still hungry, you might eat more, but if you're feeling depressed and looking for warmth, take a moment to consider your motives. Assessing your appetite and emotional state will avoid over-eating. Stop comforts like white bread and processed sugars. These foods actually cover negative emotions and cannot satisfy you until the meal is finished. You need to drink plenty of water during your meal. Recognize when you're complete and stop.

Finally, if you feed mentally, forgive yourself. If you keep thinking negatively about yourself, you're just accepting more tension and the opportunity to eat emotionally. Bad eating habits take years to establish and are uncorrectable overnight. Work for small goals and reward yourself when you enjoy something other than food.

Weight Loss Hypnosis and Controlling Emotional Eating Behaviors

Trauma and Stress

When a certain type of trauma or stress occurs in your life, many people become weighty. Divorce, death, and even unstable families and friends make many people feel relaxed feeding. Also, after stress, your emotional eating patterns are in place, and your relaxation is a natural pattern for you. One of the main goals of hypnosis of weight loss is to retrain the brain to overcome these ingrained behaviors.

Emotional Hunger

This emotional appetite is not just due to stress and trauma. Emotional hunger also leads to adolescence, events that arise with peers, and learned behavior. Most overweight people eat to relieve the pain or fill a hole in life. It feels so good to eat, and sometimes you feel guided by food when everything else is out of control. Hypnosis in weight loss aims to remove these mental causes so that you do not consume foods.

True Physical Hunger

Many people have forgotten what real physical hunger is due to emotional eating habits. When you clear your mind of these negative learned habits, it is easy to know when you are hungry. It is a slow phase, and true hunger does not just strike you out of the blue. You can feel lightheaded and lethargic when your stomach sounds rumbling; this is because your brain is signaling that it is hungry. If you get these signals, it means that the time has come to eat and avoid starvation. However, talking about true hunger, it is hard to recognize these emotional stimuli. So, it is a must turn to a method that will help you quickly!

Weight Loss Hypnosis Could Be the Key

Hypnosis of weight loss is an effective treatment that can help you to eradicate mental deprivation and emotional eating patterns for good from your life. You can go beyond computational models that have held you back for many years by simply getting into a relaxed state and listening to audio files that help you reframe your thought. Would it not be nice to reprogram your mind and body in another way to manage stress and emotional eating? Wouldn't it feel wonderful if you could act differently seamlessly so that you can really accomplish your objectives?

Beliefs and How They Affect Weight Loss

Does your conviction hold you back? There are several schools of thinking regarding a belief. But ultimately, a belief is what we really "think" or "learn." The negative side of a belief is that our life experiences shape all our values, from childhood on. Some of us heard derogatory comments from those around us when we grew up, and people might have said stuff like "you've just got big bones" or "being in your family overweight flies." We may have believed some of them, even without realizing it. A conviction isn't simply about "knowing" to be true. We can "thin" and make it a belief.

The meaning of "belief" is somewhat hazy. Beliefs are learned but can be mixed with our own hands. This is one reason the word belief has so many schools of thought.

Applying Belief Change to Weight Loss

Having a changeable belief unlocks the possibility of using the knowledge to lose weight. This brings up belief's "strength" issue. If we believe enough to do something, we're motivated to do it. It doesn't matter how our views have become our values; as long as we know, they're all changing. Everything our values belong to us, no-one else. It's up to us to act and change those values we're no longer comfortable with.

Changing Your Belief System

If we change our system of values, we change ourselves. Believe it or not (no pun intended), once people believed the planet was flat and if you sailed too far to see you'd fall off the bottom, nowadays we'd laugh our socks off if anyone asked us. That's the funny thing about beliefs, especially old beliefs, is they can harm us more than they can support us-if we let them. We will remain in our old behavior patterns because we don't think we can do anything else.

It's a self-fulfilling prophecy: if you imagine what you've always thought you're doing what you've always done, then you get what you've always got.

Ask yourself, what would I need to believe to be real to lose weight?

Understand that your values impact your life tremendously is fine, but when you take steps to change them, you will make incredible improvements in your weight to life.

This is an exercise to help you change your beliefs.

- Can you think of a belief that you know really, for instance, I'm a good driver? When you can't believe in a belief, ask when you think the day follows the night?

- Have you got an image, a feeling, or a sound? Which qualities did you experience in the picture, feeling, or sound?

- Think of a small conviction that you want to change. Take the characteristics of the belief that you know to be real and add them with the belief you want to alter.

- Make an image of the idea that you want to alter light, big, three-dimensional, bring it right before you. Now enter the note of the image; what's different?

CHAPTER 11:

Strong Weight Loss Affirmations for Woman

George taught Bonnie a hundred useful positive affirmations for weight loss and to keep her motivated. She chose the ones that she wanted to build in her program and used them every day. Bonnie was losing weight very slowly, which bothered her very much. She thought she was going in the wrong direction and was about to give up, but George told her not to worry because it was a completely natural speed. It takes time for the subconscious to collate all the information and start working according to her conscious will. Besides, her body remembered the fast weight loss, but her subconscious remembered her emotional damage, and now it is trying to prevent it. In reality, after some months of hard work, she started to see the desired results. She weighed 74 kilos (163 lbs.).

***

According to dietitians, the success of dieting is greatly influenced by how people talk about lifestyle changes for others and themselves.

The use of "I should" or "I must" should be avoided whenever possible. Anyone who says, "I shouldn't eat French fries," or "I have to get a bite of chocolate" will feel that they have no control over the events. Instead, if you say "I prefer" to leave the food, you will feel more power and less guilt. The term "dieting" should be avoided. Proper nutrition is as simple as a permanent lifestyle change. For example, the correct wording is, "I've changed my eating habits" or "I'm eating healthier."

Why Diets Are Fattening

The body needs fat. Our body wants to live, so it stores fat. Removing this amount of fat from the body is not an easy task as the body protects against weight loss. During starvation, our bodies switch to a "saving flame," burning fewer calories to avoid starving. Those who are starting to lose weight are usually optimistic, as, during the first week, they may experience 1-3 kg (2-7 lbs.) of weight loss, which validates their efforts and suffering. Their body, however, has deceived them very well because it actually does not want to break down fat. Instead, it begins to break down muscle tissue. At the beginning of dieting, our bodies burn sugar and protein, not fat. Burned sugar removes a lot of water out of the body; that's why we experience amazing results on the scale. It should take about seven days for our body to switch to fat burning. Then our body's alarm bell rings. Most diets have a sad end: reducing your metabolic rate to a lower level—Meaning that if you only eat a little more afterward, you regain all the weight you have lost previously. After dieting, the body will make special efforts to store fat for the next impending famine. What to do to prevent such a situation?

We must understand what our soul needs. Those who really desire to have success must first and foremost change their spiritual foundation. It is important to pamper our souls during a period of weight loss. All overweight people tend to rag on themselves for eating forbidden food, "I overate again. My willpower is so weak!" If you have ever tried to lose weight, you know these thoughts very well.

Imagine a person very close to you who has gone through a difficult time while making mistakes from time to time. Are we going to scold or try to help and motivate them? If we really love them, we will instead comfort them and try to convince them to continue. No one tells their best friend that they are weak, ugly, or bad just because they are struggling with their weight. If you wouldn't say it to your friend, don't do so to yourself either! Let us be aware of this: during weight loss, our soul needs peace and support. Realistic thinking is more useful than disaster theory. If you are generally a healthy consumer, eat some goodies sometimes because of their delicious taste and to pamper your soul.

I'll give you a list of a hundred positive affirmations you can use to reinforce your weight loss. I'll divide them into main categories based on the most typical situations for which you would need confirmation. You can repeat all of them whenever you need to, but you can also choose the ones that are more suitable for your circumstances. If you prefer to listen to them during meditation, you can record them with a piece of sweet relaxing music in the background.

General affirmations to reinforce your wellbeing:

- I'm grateful that I woke up today. Thank you for making me happy today.

- Today is a perfect day. I meet nice and helpful people, whom I treat kindly.

- Every new day is for me. I live to make myself feel good. Today I just pick good thoughts for myself.

- Something wonderful is happening to me today.

- I feel good.

- I am calm, energetic, and cheerful.

- My organs are healthy.

- I am satisfied and balanced.

- I live in peace and understanding with everyone.

- I listen to others with patience.

- In every situation, I find the good.

- I accept and respect myself and my fellow human beings.

- I trust myself; I trust my inner wisdom.

Do you often scold yourself? Then repeat the following affirmations frequently:

- I forgive myself.

- I'm good to myself.

- I motivate myself over and over again.

- I'm doing my job well.

- I care about myself.

- I am doing my best.

- I am proud of myself for my achievements.

- I am aware that sometimes I have to pamper my soul.

- I remember that I did a great job this week.

- I deserved this small piece of candy.

- I let go of the feeling of guilt.

- I release the blame.

- Everyone is imperfect. I accept that I am too.

If you feel pain when you choose to avoid delicious food, then you need to motivate yourself with affirmations such as:

- I am motivated and persistent.

- I control my life and my weight.

- I'm ready to change my life.

- Changes make me feel better.

- I follow my diet with joy and cheerfulness.

- I am aware of my amazing capacities.

- I am grateful for my opportunities.

- Today I'm excited to start a new diet.

- I always keep in mind my goals.

- I imagine myself as slim and beautiful as I want.

- Today I am happy to have the opportunity to do what I have long been postponing.

- I possess the energy and will to go through my diet.

- I prefer to lose weight instead of wasting time on momentary pleasures.

Here you can find affirmations that help you to change harmful convictions and blockages:

- I see my progress every day.

- I listen to my body's messages.

- I'm taking care of my health.

- I eat healthy food.

- I love who I am.

- I love how life supports me.

- A good parking space, coffee, conversation, it's all for me today.

- It feels good to be awake because I can live in peace, health, love.

- I'm grateful that I woke up. I take a deep breath of peace and tranquility.

- I love my body. I love being served by me.

- I eat by tasting every flavor of the food.

- I am aware of the benefits of healthy food.

- I enjoy eating healthy food and being fitter every day.

- I feel energetic because I eat well.

Many people are struggling with being overweight because they don't move enough. The very root of this issue can be a refusal to do exercises due to negative biases in our minds.

We can overcome these beliefs by repeating the following affirmations:

- I like moving because it helps my body burn fat.

- Each time I exercise, I am getting closer to having a beautiful, tight shapely body.

- It's a very uplifting feeling of being able to climb up to 100 steps without stopping.

- It's easier to have an excellent quality of life if I move.

- I like the feeling of returning to my home tired but happy after a long winter walk.

- Physical exercises help me have a longer life.

- I am proud to have better fitness and agility.

- I feel happier thanks to the happiness hormone produced by exercise.

- I feel full thanks to the enzymes that produce a sense of fullness during physical exercises.

- I am aware even after exercise, my muscles continue to burn fat, and so I lose weight while resting.

- I feel more energetic after exercises.

- My goal is to lose weight; therefore, I exercise.

- 66. I am motivated to exercise every day.

- I lose weight while I exercise.

Now, I am going to give you a list of generic affirmations that you can build in your program:

- I'm glad I'm who I am.

- Today, I read articles and watch movies that make me feel positive about my diet progress.

- I love it when I'm happy.

- I take a deep breath and exhale my fears.

- Today I do not want to prove my truth, but I want to be happy.

- I am strong and healthy. I'm fine, and I'm getting better.

- I am happy today because whatever I do, I find joy in it.

- I pay attention to what I can become.

- I love myself and am helpful to others.

- I accept what I cannot change.

- I am happy that I can eat healthy food.

- I am happy that I have been changing my life with my new healthy lifestyle.

- Today I do not compare myself to others.

- I accept and support who I am and turn to myself with love.

- Today I can do anything for my improvement.

- I'm fine. I'm happy for life. I love who I am. I'm strong and confident.

- I am calm and satisfied.

- Today is perfect for me to exercise and to be healthy.

- I have decided to lose weight, and I am strong enough to follow my will.

- I love myself, so I want to lose weight.

- I am proud of myself because I follow my diet program.

- I see how much stronger I am.

- I know that I can do it.

- It is not my past, but my present that defines me.

- I am grateful for my life.

- I am grateful for my body because it collaborates well with me.

- Eating healthy foods supports me in getting the best nutrients I need to be in the best shape.

- I eat only healthy foods, and I avoid processed foods.

- I can achieve my weight loss goals.

- All cells in my body are fit and healthy, and so am I.

- I enjoy staying healthy and sustaining my ideal weight.

- I feel that my body is losing weight right now.

- I care about my body by exercising every day.

CHAPTER 12:

How to Eliminate Cravings

Anyone who wants to lose weight faces the worst enemy, which is hunger and appetite. This is also felt as food cravings for different food types such as sweet, healthy, or, even worse, unhealthy foods such as chocolate; hence the word "chocoholic."

First of all, it's these food cravings that make you overweight, but the cravings are further magnified when you go on a diet, as it has been shown that when you don't take enough calories, food cravings are intensified cravings for high-calorie sweet and fatty foods particularly.

As a consequence, when you eat, you are much more likely to pick something extremely calorific, thus undoing your low-calorie regime's weight-loss gain.

It is further exacerbated by the fact that when you lose weight, your body tries to resist it (a survival mechanism that developed when food became scarce) and slows down your metabolism while increasing food cravings, particularly cravings for high carbohydrate, high fat, and high sugar foods.

All these physiological factors combine to make it very difficult for the dieter to make lower-calorie food choices and sustain weight-loss.

Indeed, the widely heard phrases of "food cravings" and "food addiction" or "chocoholic" have become phrases precisely because the perception is similar to drug addicts. The compulsion to eat, particularly high-carb and high-fat foods, can be stronger than heroin addicts' compulsions.

The disastrously low diet success rates are further evidence of the difficulties of avoiding food cravings. In five years, 95% of dieters recover their weight and more. For a long time, the vast majority of us are unable to combat them effectively, making our weight-loss goals seem unattainable.

I personally noticed that, while I know the best foods to fill me with fewer calories, and I tried to include as many of these types of foods as possible in my diet, I still encountered carbohydrate cravings and sugar products that took me over my weight loss calorie cap.

I often found that I sometimes just didn't have the time to prepare lower-calorie alternatives, or that lower-calorie alternatives were just not available (e.g., like eating "on the run"), or that I actually liked meals that were higher in calories and didn't consider lower-calorie options. For example, with my eggs and sandwiches, I really prefer buttered toast!

Wouldn't it be so much easier if we could take a pill that would allow us to consume more carbohydrate foods without the caloric after-effects (i.e., weight gain)?

Well, after my extensive and thorough study into the best weight-loss methods and critical review, I'm sure there are a variety of supplements that make the weight-loss process easier.

One of the most exciting supplements I tested is a drug that helps to reduce the absorption of dietary carbohydrates.

It's all good, healthy, value-for-money, side-effect-free, efficient for long-term use, and has a powerful weight-loss-assisting performance. And, most significantly, for the customer, scientific data can be checked out to support their claims of efficacy.

Tips from Hypnosis Weight Loss Programs

Weight management is one of the main factors in ensuring you lead a happy, safe lifestyle. When you're an emotional eater, it's harder to regulate your weight. There are many different nutritional areas that lead to weight management, making it easier to avoid emotional eating and safely lose weight.

- The first thing to bear in mind is the addictive effect that food has on you. You may encounter cravings that often feel uncontrollable, and you can feel like getting food addiction, just like a smoker is addicted to smoking.

- The trick is to control your emotions and feelings properly and train your brain not to respond to unpleasant or uncomfortable feelings by simply consuming food (your preferred brain drug) to calm down.

- Dieting kills your metabolism and can potentially make you weigh. In reality, dieting works only short-term and lowers your fragile self-esteem.

- Change the way you think; women appear to think differently from an overweight or obese male. They don't add emotion to food and don't use food to self-medicate and feel better.

- Learn alternative techniques for de-stressing and calming rather than eating.

Recognize You're Eating Triggers

Eviting or avoiding the food you know causes you to weigh and satisfy your cravings, and emotional eating is typically snack foods, cakes, cookies, etc. I also test for food allergy or food sensitivity. Even healthy foods can lead you to food addiction and weight gain.

The easiest way to lose weight will be removing something very common from your diet and releasing years of unnecessary fat exercise at the gym. Remember, brain and body exercises such as yoga, Pilates, or even walking in a nice park will do wonders for your mind, self-esteem, and body.

Relax More

Take some time to reconnect with yourself. Most people don't know how to relax properly and think it's enough sitting in front of the Screen-it's not. Study some basic meditation techniques to relax completely.

Don't Compare Yourself to Others

When you're losing weight, it's important not to compare your weight to those around you. If you're unhappy with your weight, comparing yourself to the skinny girls you see in magazines or on television that prolong your recovery process by adjusting your lifestyle habits with eating, exercise, and mind control, you'll find it much easier to stop emotional eating and lose the weight you want much faster and longer-term. When you've learned techniques to regulate eating causes and cravings, emotional eating will end.

In a person who controls their emotions and has more positive ways of coping with negative feelings, emotional eating cannot thrive-it's unlikely. Before you know it, you'll eat intuitively and be rid of emotional eating and excess body fat for good.Are you sick of getting the same old weight loss advice? Looking for some fast tips to help empower yourself to stop the holiday weight gain? Why not follow to learn about some fast, safe weight loss tips?

- **Eliminate five pounds before a major case:** If you're usually in good health but want a few pounds off to look your best before a major event like New Year's Eve or a class reunion, one of the best ways to do it is to clean your body.

Miss bread and pasta the week before, eat plenty of raw vegetables and salads, keep lean protein in the mix, and drink at least eight ounces of water a day. You won't only end up slimmer; you'll feel 100% more confident and safer.

Actually, your weight fluctuates during the day, so your best bet is never on the scale, only when medically appropriate. Losing five pounds will make you feel fantastic quickly, but the dieting coaster can also start. If you've ever taken the trip, won't you ever get off the diet roller coaster?

- **Weight without diet:** It's better than you thought. Dieting generates fault habit. Skip diets and count. Expect to eat regular, balanced meals three times a day, 4 hours apart.

- **Know it's a workout:** A brisk one-mile stroll, half an hour of dancing, or chasing the kids around in a tag game. The trick is to keep it at first for 20 to 30 minutes and then add more every day after a week.

- **Right-start your day:** Cutting calories during vacations also means missing meals. Unfortunately, this slows down the metabolism to speed it up. Don't miss breakfast while you're trying to lose weight, and don't opt for "nutrition bars" comfort. Instead, give your body a raw pick-me-up of fresh fruit, and protein, and whole-grain staying power. Some of the favorite breakfasts are a fried egg or microwave scrambled egg, a bowl of whole-grain cereal with fresh fruit, melon, or peaches.

You get the lean protein that lets you stay alert, building the muscle that burns the fat, the sugar that your brain craves, the carbohydrates it requires to work on and adding antioxidant vitamins to help it stay on track and recover.

- **Take daily high-quality dietary supplements:** There's no alternative for eating a balanced mix of all ingredients, but skimping on the basics is all too easy when attempting to lose weight. Make sure the body doesn't lack the nutrients it needs because you cut calories. A healthy dietary supplement includes vitamins and antioxidants to optimize the machinery in your cells.

  A broad multivitamin would provide minimum recommended daily amounts of vitamins A, B6, B12, C, E, and K. While at it, get out in the sun at least ten minutes a day to help the body produce the vitamin D it needs. Alternatively, a lot of work has shown that most people have low vitamin D, and they can also take vitamin D supplements.

- **Eat vegetables, particularly lettuce:** Yet don't rely on iceberg lettuce or salads. Seek braised, steamed, or grilled for something different from the regular salad.

- **Set an optimistic or concrete target.** Instead of thinking or talking about how to "lose 5 pounds," plan to weigh your weight. For example, take your current weight, subtract 5, and believe you already weigh that amount.

  If you have difficulty believing this, learning to use hypnosis will help you improve yourself safely and comfortably. A trained hypnotist using a validated hypnosis training technique with real client outcomes will show you how in a comprehensive weight loss program.

- **Eliminate failure habit:** Weight loss failure due to past failures. It induces a pattern of disappointment or "disappointment presumption" for new behaviors.

One of my favorite quotes from Dr. Stephen Covey is, "You can't think about the situation you've acted in!" Just taking action on these tips can create significant improvements in attitude, weight, and shape. What do you do if you make the above moves, but you don't lose weight?

Hypnosis and other self-help methods can be very helpful in improving your behavior. Unfortunately, you can't know from reading a novel. Only a live, individualized learning system may yield long-term results.

CHAPTER 13:

Weight Loss Hypnosis Program

Many of us battle to discover success in the very things we long for daily. There are different techniques to reach the things that we want, but not all things work for one individual as it would for another. A displayed strategy for success for many individuals that require little exertion is meditation. Obviously, from the get-go, it very well may be hard to start this procedure. With the correct steps taken and a readiness to go at something new, you can get the things you've been yearning for with the abilities that already exist inside your mind. The ideal way to digest the media we are about to present to you is by doing such through a book. At the point when you hear something repeated to you, your mind will be significantly more prone to recollect the information you're presented with.

But you will also focus and concentrate rather than attempting to make sense of the words you're reading. It's easier for your brain to take what it hears faster if it saw the information. This is how many individuals learn and keep information. Allowing another person to introduce this to you through an audiobook will also be better because that person will do it at the correct pace. If you attempt to read to yourself, you may finish far too quickly than how we are introducing the information to you. By allowing another person to take the lead and pace things out for you, it will be easier to take in the media as it ought to be. Tune in to this when you are home and in a safe area. It is enticing to tune in on the train as you're commuting to work, or even in the car, but we don't always know how we may react to hypnosis and meditation. You may be excessively calm and not have the option to drive appropriately, or you could even fall asleep when hypnotized. Nothing too dangerous can happen to you as long as you stay home, or if nothing else, in a place where falling asleep is safe. Meditation is self-coordinated.

Let's now start! 5, 4, 3, 2, 1. I am going to guide you through different hypnosis now. This one is focused on weight loss. I am going to help you find the results that you have always wanted, all by unlocking the things in your brain needed to start this process. First, make sure that you are sitting somewhere comfortably. A metronome might help regulate your breathing as well.

First, start by placing your hand on your stomach. As you do this, feel the body that exists underneath. It's not the one you want right now, but it's the one that you have. As you breathe in, feel your stomach expand.

As you let that air out, feel your stomach flatten. Now, count to five with me as you breathe in. One, two, three, four, five. Count to six as you breathe out. Hold for an extra second because I want you to feel your stomach flatten. Become aware of how different your body can change.

Now, sit with your hands somewhere comfortable, focusing only on your closed eyes. Keep breathing in and out, again, noticing the differences that you can simply feel in your body through your stomach muscles. The things that our bodies are capable of are pretty incredible. Knowing all the abilities, we have with them can be very enlightening.

When we are in tune with our bodies and attached to all of the things that they can do, it's going to be much easier to make sure that we are making healthy decisions that are best for them.

Now, slowly let your mind drift somewhere relaxing. Pick a place in nature. Maybe it's a forest, a beach, or a large grassy field. Wherever it is, I want you to envision this. Now, I'm going to count to ten again, and as I do, your mind is going black. One, two three, four, five, six, seven, eight, nine, ten.

Now, you see nothing but black. As you focus on nothing, a small light emerges, and you see it starting to grow. As it does, you become more and more relaxed, still feeling the air enter and exit your body. The light keeps going, and before you know it, it is pouring all over your body.

You suddenly realize that you aren't thinking about this place in nature; you are there. As you look around, there is green surrounding you. The blue sky emerges through the leafy green trees, and you can feel the warm sun start to warm your skin.

A cool breeze comes over your body, and you feel the freshness through your hair. You are not afraid of being alone in this place in nature. It is something that you have been waiting for. This is what you deserve.

You start to walk forward, not going anywhere in particular. As you take each step, you start to see a small building in the distance. You are slowly walking, feeling your body relax. You feel light, fresh, healthy. Something about the way you feel now is different than how you did before.

The building is right in front of you now, and you take it upon yourself to walk in. as you open the door, light pours onto you, and you suddenly feel even more rejuvenated. The building is air-conditioned, and you can tell that it is fresh and new. You aren't sure where you are, but it doesn't matter. No one seems to be there, but you are not afraid to be alone. As you walk in, you see a mirror standing right in front of you.

At first, you are afraid to look into it. There might be a person looking back at you that you do not want to see. Something is telling you that it is time to look into this mirror, however. As you walk up to it, you are shocked to see the person that is looking back at you. This is a person that you don't recognize at first. She is healthy. She is smiling. Their skin is clear, and her hair is radiant. She is fit, and you can tell that she is working out. The more you look at her, the more you realize that this is you. This is the version that you have been waiting for.

You have had visions in the past of what it might look like if you were to finally decide to go through with your weight loss journey. Now, you are here. You are looking into the mirror and seeing a person that you have been hoping for all along. You are happy and healthy. You are confident, and you are excited.

As you look into the mirror, you suddenly remember all that it took to get there. There were moments where you thought that you couldn't do it. There were times when the only thing that felt right was for you to give up. There were many obstacles in your way, but you finally had the courage to fight through them and get what you wanted.

As you look at your legs, you see that they are strong. They carried you for your entire life, helping you get places that you would never have imagined. You can see the outline of your muscles in them, so strong and sleek. As you move up, you see the flat stomach that you have always wanted.

You might still have a few stretch marks, but they are there as a reminder of how much you worked for your health. You fought for yourself for your body. You went through things that others aren't able to do on their own. You see this in your torso. All the food that looked so appetizing that you said "no" to shows in your flat stomach now. Every time you chose something healthy instead of something simply tasty is making itself present in your body.

As you look into the mirror, you see that your chest is strong as well. This healthy chest protects your heart, and you can feel it working well as it sends blood throughout your body. You are feeling energized, correct, fulfilled, and happy. Finally, you see your shoulders and arms. These are so strong and have also helped to carry you so far.

You look at them from your fingers to your neck, toned and supporting the rest of your body. Though you have seen all of the important changes throughout the rest of your body, the thing that is most important is how large your smile is now. Your cheeks are stretched to show the radiance that has always existed inside of you and can finally be present now.

It feels so good to know that you look this good, but what is even better than that is the fact that you are so comfortable with your body. Throughout your weight loss, you learned how to take care of yourself in a healthy way so that you will be able to keep the weight off for a long time. There were moments when all you wanted was a specific body, but right here, smiling into the mirror, you know now that the most important thing is that you are happy.

It is time now for me to bring you out of the hypnosis. When I count to ten, you are going to be back into the present world, ready to start your journey. One, two, three, four, five, six, seven, eight, nine, ten.

CHAPTER 14:

Deep Sleep Meditation

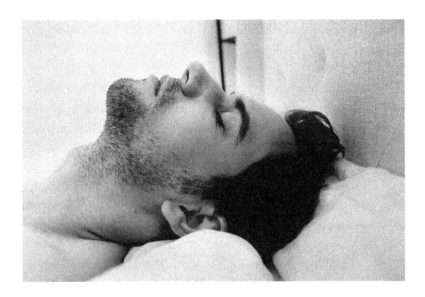

Deep Sleep Meditation

One of the best ways to become relaxed and find the peace needed for better sleep is through the use of a visualization technique. For this, you will want to ensure that you are in a thoroughly relaxing and comfortable place. This reading will help you more centered on the moment, alleviate anxiety, and wind down before bed.

Listen to it as you are falling asleep, whether it's at night or if you are simply taking a nap. Ensure the lighting is right and remove all other distractions that will keep you from becoming completely relaxed.

Meditation for a Full Night's Sleep

You are lying in a completely comfortable position right now. Your body is well-rested, and you are prepared to drift deeply into sleep. The deeper you sleep, the healthier you feel when you wake up.

Your eyes are closed, and the only thing that you are responsible for now is falling asleep. There isn't anything you should be worried about other than becoming well-rested. You are going to be able to do this through this guided meditation into another world.

It will be the transition between your waking life and a place where you will fall into a deep and heavy sleep. You are becoming more relaxed and ready to fall into a trance-like state where you can drift into healthy sleep.

Start by counting down slowly. Use your breathing in fives to help you become more and more asleep.

You are now more and more relaxed and prepared for a night of deep and heavy sleep. You are drifting away, faster and faster, deeper and deeper, closer and closer to a heavy sleep. You see nothing as you let your mind wander.

You are not fantasizing about anything. You are not worried about what has happened today or even farther back in your past. You are not afraid of what might be there going forward. You are not fearful of anything in the future that is causing you panic.

You are highly aware of this moment that everything will be OK. Nothing matters but your breathing and your relaxation. Everything in front of you is peaceful. You are filled with serenity, and you exude calmness. You only think about what is happening in the present moment where you are becoming more and more at peace.

Your mind is blank. You see nothing but black. You are fading faster and faster, deeper and deeper, further and further. You are getting close to being completely relaxed, but right now, you are OK with sitting here peacefully.

You aren't rushing to sleep because you need to wind down before bed. You don't want to go to bed with anxious thoughts and have nightmares about the things you fear. The only thing that you concern yourself with at this moment is getting friendly and relaxed before it's time to start to sleep.

You see nothing in front of you other than a small white light. That light becomes a bit bigger and bigger. As it grows, you start to see that you are inside a vehicle. You are lying on your bed; everything around you is still there. Only when you look up, you see that there is a large open window, with several computers and wheels out in front of you.

You realize that you are in a spaceship floating peacefully through the sky. It is on auto-pilot, and there is nothing that you have to worry about as you are floating up in this spaceship. You look out above you and see that the night sky is gorgeous than you ever could have imagined.

All that surrounds you is nothing but beauty. Bright stars are twinkling against a black backdrop. You can make out some of the planets. They are all different than you would ever have imagined. Some are bright purple; others are blue. There are detailed swirls and stripes that you didn't know were there.

You relax and feel yourself floating up in this space. When you are here, everything seems so small. You still have problems back home on Earth, but they are so distant that they are almost not real. Some issues make you feel as though the world is ending, but now that the entire universe is still doing fine, no matter what might be happening in your life. You are not concerned with any issues right now.

You are soaking up all that is around you. You are so far separated from Earth, and it's crazy to think about just how much space is out there for you to explore. You are relaxed, looking around. There are shooting stars all in the distance. There are floating rocks passing by your ship. You are floating around, feeling dreamier and dreamier.

You are passing over Earth again, getting close to going back home. You will be sent right back into your room, falling more heavily with each breath you take back into sleep. You are getting closer and closer to drifting away.

You pass over the Earth and look down to see all of the beauty that exists. The green and blue swirl together, white clouds above that make such an interesting pattern. Everything below looks like a painting. It does not seem real.

You get closer and closer, floating so delicately in your small space ship. The ride is not bumpy. It is not bothering you.

You are floating over the city now. You see, random lights flicker on. It doesn't look like a map anymore, like when you are so high above.

You are looking down and seeing that gentle lights still flash here and there, but for the most part, the city is winding down. Everyone is drifting faster and faster to sleep. You are getting closer and closer to your home. You see that everything is peaceful below you. The sun will rise again, and tomorrow will start. For now, the only thing you can do is prepare and rest for what might come.

You are more and more relaxed now, drifting further and further into sleep.

You still focused on your breathing; it is becoming slower and slower. You are close to drifting away to sleep now.

When we reach one, you will drift off deep into sleep.

How Meditation Helps Weight Loss

Meditation is known to be a useful tool for weight loss. It aligns the unconscious mind with the conscious mind to facilitate changes that we want to make in our behaviors. Such modifications may include avoiding unhealthy foods by altering them with healthier foods. Your unconscious mind must become engaged in the change process because it is where the weight-gaining, poor habits such as emotional eating. Through meditation, you will be able to become more aware of your surroundings and will be able to overcome your unhealthy habits.

But there is even a more immediate effect of mediation. It can reduce the level of stress hormones in the body. Hormones like cortisol give the body signal to store more calories. If you have high levels of cortisol moving through your system, it will be challenging to cut down weight even if you are eating healthy foods. Most of us stressed in most cases, but it takes only 25 minutes of meditation three times in a row to reduce the effects of stress.

In 2016, a study conducted by Texas Tech University found that increased relaxation, attention, body-mind awareness, calmness, and brain activity resulted from just a few sessions of meditation. The study also suggested that your self-control could increase with daily meditation. The researchers found that the brain is most affected by reflection, which means that with a few minutes of meditation, you will pass by that ice cream when feeling stressed.

How to Start Meditating for Weight Loss

Even without training, anyone who has a body and mind can practice meditation. For most of us, the most challenging aspect of meditation is getting time. You can start with as little as 8 to 10 minutes a day.

Ensure that you can access a quiet place for meditation. If you have children or other people around you, you may need to squeeze time

EXTREME WEIGHT LOSS HYPNOSIS

when they are not awake or leave the house to avoid distractions. You may even practice your mediation while in the shower.

Once you are in a place of silence, take a comfortable position. You can either lie down or sit in an area that makes you feel at ease.

Start meditating by putting your focus on your breath. Watch the way your stomach or chest rises and falls. Feel the air that you breathe in and out of your mouth. Listen keenly to the sounds around you. This should be done for 2 or 3 minutes until you begin feeling relaxed.

Next, do the following steps:

- Take in a deep breath, and hold for a few seconds

- Slowly breathe out, and repeat the process

- Breathe in a natural manner

- Observe how your breath enters your nostrils, influence the movement of your chest, and move your stomach

- Continue focusing on the way you breathe in and out for about 8 to 10 minutes

- Your mind may begin to wonder, which is a regular occurrence. Just acknowledge this and return your attention to the process

- As you wrap up, reflect on your thoughts and recognize how you can quickly bring your mind together.

CHAPTER 15:

Using Hypnosis to Change Eating Habits

Habits rule much of your everyday activities, especially your food and exercise habits. In addition to hypnosis, paying attention to your habits is an important step in weight loss because your habits dictate whether you will adapt your eating habits to match what goals you need to make. Forty percent of what you do each day is habitual, so if you don't pay attention to your habits, you're missing an important chunk of your behavior and failing to make it align with your goals. If you want to lose weight, some, but not all, habits will have to change.

Because so much of our life is ruled by habits, you need to determine what your worst dietary and exercise habits are. For one week or so, keep track of your eating and exercise patterns, especially pay attention to times when you mindlessly eat or emotionally eat. Track what you eat and why you are eating it. Also, track the kinds of exercises you do and for how long. During this process, you can begin to pick up on some of your habits that may not be initially apparent when you try to pinpoint the habits you want to change. Some of your habits may be obvious from the start, but others will be more covert. Once you have discovered your habits, find ways to replace your bad habits with good ones to encourage the changes that you want in your life.

Replacing unhealthy habits can be hard because habits are so ingrained in you that you often don't notice that you are doing them, but focusing on creating good habits instead of bad ones can brighten your attitude and make it easier to stick to your plan. As you replace your bad habits, create habits that you enjoy and that give you enrichment. If you don't like celery, don't replace your chip eating habit with a celery eating habit. Try carrots and hummus or rice cakes. There are hundreds of good alternatives to any bad habit, so find ones that work for you and don't make you feel like you're completely losing.

Don't try to change everything at once. Start one or a couple of habits at a time. If you try to do too much habit-changing at once, your brain will struggle to focus and keep up with all the changes that you need to be making. Integrate your new habits gradually so that it's not a shock to your system. You have plenty of time to complete your transformation, so don't rush it. You wouldn't want a contractor rushing to build your house just to get it done, and you'd be angry if he did a half-hearted job, so you need to take your time with your weight loss and do it the proper and effective way. If you can manage to break more than a couple of habits at once, throw in some more habits to break, but as always, know your limits.

Reward yourself when you do well. Encourage yourself whenever you find yourself not making your bad habits. For example, if you're able to make it twenty-one days without mindlessly eating in front of the TV, promise yourself that you can go get your nails done or that you can buy a pair of new shoes. Make it worth your while. Giving yourself things to look forward to is a huge motivation and puts your mind on what you can gain instead of letting it fixate on what you're losing. It may be hard to see this now, but by the end of your journey, you won't feel like you've lost anything. You'll merely feel balanced and like you've gained a new chance to be the person you want to be.

Get your loved ones involved in your weight loss journey and allow them to be part of your plans. Maybe one of your friends also wants to lose weight or achieve new fitness goals. Going on this journey together can be an important bonding experience, and not having to go through the process alone makes it significantly easier. So, if you find a friend who is willing and able, be each other's support system and hold each other accountable. Even if they don't diet with you, lean on your family and friends to be your cheerleaders, and push you to be your best self even when you are feeling discouraged.

Get rid of things that might encourage bad habits. If you're a chip junkie, limit how many chips you keep in your house. When you have habits that you want to get rid of, the best thing you can do is keep the temptations far away. That way, when you'd normally or habitually reach for the bag of chips, you have to consciously become aware of the fact that you don't have any chips. From there, you are given a choice to teach yourself to look for something else, or you have to make a conscious effort to get those chips. When you have to consciously do something, that's helping you resist the habitual draw because you have to stop and think about what you are doing.

Use visualization to see yourself as the person you want to be. Visualization is a superb tool to help you imagine your goals and then achieve them. Imagine yourself where you want to be one year from now. Think of how you'll look, but also imagine how you will feel. Think of how differently you'll move when you lose weight. Think of all the obstacles you'll no longer have to face. Think of the freedom you will feel and the weight that will be lifted from your shoulders. Imagine yourself as calm, stress-free, and thinner. Each day, it can help to go to bed and wake up, visualizing the person you'd like to be.

Be aware of the hardship and the payoff. Always keep the payoff in your mind and remind yourself why you want to change. If you don't keep what you want in the forefront of your mind, your dreams will get lost in the chaos of your head. The hardship seems a lot worse when you think of all the amazing things that can come from that work. Challenges can also be psychologically rewarding because when you don't feel challenged, you feel bored and stagnated, which leads to restlessness and unhappiness.

Don't allow yourself to say that it's not working and give up. Be patient with yourself. If you're only a week in, and you're already starting to convince yourself that it's hopeless, then you're the problem. When you don't let yourself see the whole process through, you are failing yourself, and you are refusing to accomplish the steps you need to take to become the person you want to be. Go back and do more mental preparation until you feel ready to give this your all. Give yourself at least a month. Habits can take anywhere from twenty-one days to upwards of two months to form. Thus, if you don't stick that time out, Don't give up on your dieting plans until you've at least given a one-month effort, preferably more. If you give it that long, you'll find that it starts to get easier.

Start right away. Don't put weight loss off until tomorrow. You need to start this process right now and not let yourself run away fearfully from the things that you want to accomplish. If you don't start right away, you will keep putting your weight loss dreams off until there isn't another tomorrow. There's absolutely no reason to delay this journey. It may seem overwhelming now, but it's completely manageable for anyone willing to put the time and effort in.

Set Yourself up for Success

The ultimate goal of hypnosis and the heart of this whole book is to set yourself up for success. So many diets are bound to fail, but because this plan allows you to make permanent changes and to teach your brain to act in better ways, accordingly, you aren't set up to fail. Though, as good as this information is, the brunt of the burden of success is on you. You're the one who has to put in all the work to set yourself up for success, so take that duty seriously.

Take the time to focus on yourself. It's not selfish to want to take some special time to care for your own needs. So many people dedicated their lives to other people, and that's a noble thing, but every person also needs to care for their own needs so that they can better serve other people and feel confident about who they are. Find time to reflect on your growth and weight loss journey in addition to finding time for hypnosis. We all have busy lives, but cutting back on one TV episode a day can make an immense difference in how much you can accomplish. You deserve to feel good about yourself, so prioritize that, and you'll be able to find the time.

Be open to change. You're not going to be able to stick by your old and comfortable habits. You'll have to learn to welcome in the new and embrace the uncertainty that every new journey brings. Sometimes you will feel like you're so far out of your element, but that's a good thing! When you feel like that, you are changing and growing as a person. Don't be afraid to try new things and experiment with what you eat and what activities you do. There's no limit to how much you can learn about yourself, and of course, if you're open to change, you'll welcome the weight loss. Too many people subconsciously close themselves off to weight loss, so make a conscious effort to remain open to new information about the world and yourself.

Don't doubt yourself. Have faith in your ability to accomplish your goals. There's genuinely nothing to stand in your way of success. You hold all the power in this transformation, so if you want to do well, believing in yourself can go a long way.

Hypnotherapy can work better when you're in the right headspace to do it, which is we have emphasized getting into the right headspace for hypnosis and learning about what hypnosis fundamentally is. With all the information you've read so far, you should feel ready to set yourself up for success and finally dive into the actual hypnosis. There will still be plenty of mental work ahead, but now that you've created the mental foundation, you can handle all of it with grace and relative ease. Your mind has amazing powers, the ones you only need to channel to do it well. Never question that you can make changes that will last for the rest of your life.

CHAPTER 16:

Step-by-Step Hypnotherapy for Weight Loss

S tart by taking a deep breath in, then let it out slowly. Make sure that you are seated comfortably and that you are somewhere safe where you can relax for twenty minutes or so. During this session, you will ignore all daily noises like the telephone ringing, traffic sounds outside, or any other sounds except for sounds of alarm. If you hear an alarming sound, you will immediately come out of the trance state with no residual sleepiness.

Relax, take another breath in, and out. Let go of all of the stress that you are holding onto. Relax, breathe in, and out.

Start by relaxing the muscles in your feet and legs. Think of each muscle one by one and let them all just let go and relax. Feel a warmth spreading from your toes up to your calves, feel the warmth go to your thighs, and as it moves across your body, feel each muscle group that it reaches, let go and relax completely.

Relax your stomach muscles….and moving up to your chest and shoulders. Feel the warmth move up your body and relax, breathe in and out; now your neck muscles are feeling warm and relaxed. Feel all of the muscles in your face relax completely.

Imagine yourself at the top of an escalator. As you step onto the escalator, you realize that you are passing numbers on white signs on the way down. The first number is 10. As you pass each number, you will fall deeper and deeper into a relaxed state. Take another deep breath in….9, the escalator is moving you slowly forward and down…8, you are becoming more and more relaxed each time you pass a number…7, relax your body completely and let go of everything….6….you reach the halfway point of the slow-moving escalator…5, you are very relaxed, now completely relaxed…4, you feel as if you are floating down the escalator becoming more and more relaxed…3….you can see the bottom, and when you reach it you will become even more deeply relaxed than you are now..2, you reach the bottom of the escalator…1, breathe in and out very relaxed now.

With each of the suggestions that I give to you, you will become more deeply relaxed than before. Each of these suggestions will stay in your subconscious, and they will be used to influence your behavior when you awake; continue to relax as each suggestion is given.

You no longer have to eat too much food to feel the good feelings about yourself that the food provides; your feelings are good as they are.

When you feel an emotion, your response is to eat. However, you don't need to do that. When you feel anxiety, you should slow down and try to find the cause. You don't need to overeat to solve anxiety. Overeating will not solve the problem; it will only make it worse. If you feel depressed, that means that it is time to spring into action. When you feel frustrated, what you have been doing may not be working, and instead of eating, try something else. If you feel stressed, you will not become less stressed by eating. Instead, try to relax and take things one by one as they come. If you feel the emotion of loneliness, try to surround yourself with people instead of food.

Eating will not satisfy these emotions. When you feel these emotions, your response will be to do something other than eating. In the future, you will find it easier to understand these emotions, and you will not feel compelled to eat. Your feelings are there to guide you through life, and each one means something different. Your response to these will no longer be to eat. Instead, you will allow each emotion to happen and then take action.

In the future, you will be free from the cycle that you have fallen into in the past. Eating will not solve any problems, even temporarily, and will only make you feel worse. Eating should only be done when you are hungry, and you should eat until you are no longer hungry. When you find yourself tempted to make large portions, you will have the willpower to say no, and you will be very satisfied with the amount you have.

When you have other emotions, they are not hunger. Those are simply emotions, and eating will not make them go away. You will remember these things when you awake. As I count up from 1, you will start to feel more awake, but still, remember all the suggestions given…2….you are coming up…3, you are starting to feel less relaxed and more alert…4, when you awake at the end of the count, you will feel refreshed and ready to continue your daily activities…5, you are more awake now…6….7….8….9….you will wake up completely refreshed on the number 10.

Self-confidence is essential to progress well in your life. Not enough confidence prevents you from going to the maximum of what you can do and from developing fully. But too much pretense of self-confidence will close the door on you. Self-confidence is, therefore, good as long as you don't go to extremes: be honest with yourself and trust yourself. How to successfully achieve this goal? With only a little practice.

Nothing is sexier than a woman who radiates confidence!

CHAPTER 17:

Hypnosis Weight Loss Practical Tips

To achieve your weight loss goals, you must be willing to let any fear and doubt you have about hypnotherapy. It is not something that you can second guess, particularly not its effectivity and results-driven orientation. It is a solution used for many different reasons, even other than weight loss. Hypnotherapy for weight loss can help you overcome a negative relationship with food, one that may have formed over a period or throughout your entire life. It is something that can present you with proper results and that you can always be sure of.

Although it is not a diet or weight loss supplement, it fulfills a similar supporting role and serves as the foundation for a more mindful lifestyle. Since the method thereof is focused on replacing old negative habits with new positive ones, it helps one to overcome challenges faced when trying to lose weight.

Both can serve you usefully whether you want to opt for a one-on-one weight loss for hypnotherapy session or listen to audiobooks online.

Before you dive into the world of hypnotherapy, you should know that there's a lot more to it than you initially thought. Much like Yoga and meditation, in general, it serves a higher purpose as it leads you on to a mindful path of physical, mental, and emotional wellness.

Tips for Weight Loss Hypnosis

- **Find the right hypnotherapist for weight loss for you.** How would you go about doing this, you may ask? Instead of going the obvious route of searching for hypnotherapists online in your area, why not ask for recommendations instead? What's better than asking a friend, family member, or acquaintance to recommend you an ethical hypnotherapist for weight loss? If no one knows or knows a hypnotherapist that is known for the outstanding jobs they perform, you may want to check with your doctor and ask for advice. They should be able to recommend a qualified and results-oriented hypnotherapist for weight loss. To ensure you have the right hypnotherapist once you've found one, be sure to check with yourself whether their consultation felt as though it was thorough, whether the hypnotherapy program was adjusted to meet your needs if there were any, and whether the practitioner was helpful and answered all of your questions. When hypnotherapists allow for space between sessions, it's also an indication that you're dealing with an ethical hypnotherapist.

- **Don't pay any attention to advertising.** We live in 2021, which means that everything we see online is taken seriously. However, it shouldn't be. People are oblivious and susceptible to accept everything they read or hear, but when it comes to advertising, not everything can be trusted. Advertising should, ever so often, be disregarded and not taken too seriously as it can be very misleading. It's always better to conduct your research before you accept that something is a sure way or not. In the case of hypnotherapy, since there are so many negative associations related to the practice, it's best to find out what's it all about yourself. As you can see from this useful set of information about hypnotherapy for weight loss, it is entirely safe and probably nothing negative that you expected it to be.

- **Get information about training, qualifications, and necessary experience.** Before you pick a hypnotherapist, you must be sure about their essential information first. Do they run their practice or operate independently? Are they certified and have a license? Ensuring that they also adhere to ethical standards, most preferably recommended by other medical physicians, you'll be assured that you are dealing with someone who knows what they are doing.

- **Before choosing one hypnotherapist, talk to several first.** Perhaps one of the best ways to find out whether a hypnotherapist is best suited for you is to speak with a few of them over a phone call first. This will take some effort, but it will be worth it in the end. You have to consider whether they can relate to you, care about your well-being, and listen to your concerns, whether they are personable, accommodating, and professional. If they tick all the boxes, then you're good to go.

- **Don't fall for any promises that may sound unrealistic.** If a hypnotist tells you that their therapy session will help you lose weight fast, don't even bother going to a single session. In reality, hypnosis for weight loss is a process that takes time. It can take anywhere between three weeks, up to three months to see your physical body change and lose weight. Since your body and mind should first adjust, you need to allow time to do so. Hypnosis for weight loss isn't a fad, nor is it a means of losing weight overnight. It's also essential to avoid hypnotherapists who suggest they will make you lose weight. Since they will only be talking during the session, what they're telling you is not true whatsoever. What you can expect from a professional and authentic hypnotherapist, however, is a professional individual who takes responsibility for helping you to get where you want to go. This person should help you access your subconscious mind with ease and help you bring it on board with a proper weight loss plan and possibly an exercise routine.

- **Is your hypnotherapist of choice multi-skilled?** Hypnosis is a terrific tool and can alter the mind's way of thinking about food, and it goes hand-in-hand with nutrition. This is something you need to consider, mainly whether your hypnotist has a good understanding of what it takes for you to lose weight sustainably and healthily. Many people who are focused on starting a weight loss journey don't necessarily know what to do or what they should eat. When looking for a hypnotherapist, look for a self-help coaching or some psychotherapy qualification, as well as a qualification/background in either nutrition or cognitive behavioral therapy.

- **Find out the time you should engage in a program.** This is quite important as hypnotherapy can become quite expensive if you're going to a professional for one-on-one sessions. If you prefer going to a professional rather than conducting the courses at your home, you can choose to spread your sessions over time to make it more affordable. Even though you may think that the meetings become less useful to achieve the overall effect, it works more effectively as your mind and body require time to adjust. Time is also needed as you change your old habits and replace them with new ones.

- **Ask your hypnotherapist if they can provide you with a program to maintain your progress at home.** A recording mainly helps to allow you to spread out sessions over time. Listening to your weight loss hypnosis recording will keep you in check and help you stay motivated and focused.

- **Ask your hypnotherapist if they can tailor-make your hypnotherapy weight loss program for you.** If they agree to it, you can expect a weight loss hypnotherapy program that is much more effective than individualized hypnosis. It offers treatments that may work better than ones that cater to everyone. Since every person is different compared to others, this makes a lot more sense. Sure, the general program will work, but a personalized one could offer you better results.

- **Ask whether your program includes an introduction session.** Starting with hypnotherapy for weight loss, you don't want to dive right into it. It's essential to take the necessary time, even if it's just an hour, to establish your needs and concerns regarding your current habits, lifestyle, and goals with your hypnotherapist. Ensuring that they care about your well-being and results instead of just taking you through the session is equally important. Taking the time to talk to your hypnotherapist and getting to know them better will help you feel more at ease and form a foundation of trust before starting with your hypnotherapy sessions.

- **Establish the costs involved before starting with your sessions.** Ensuring you know how much an initial consultation and each session fee will be another essential factor you have to consider before choosing a hypnotherapist. Considering the cost, consider an overview of their program compared to other potential weight loss programs, review the price solely based on the quality of service you'll receive, and take into account that you can spread your application over weeks instead of going to a few sessions a week.

Lastly, it would help if you viewed hypnotherapy as an investment in yourself and well-being, rather than an unnecessary expense. The context for this thought will realize once you engage in or complete your program.

CHAPTER 18:

Eating the Right Foods
Becomes Automatic

There are multiple types of diets or nutritional options, such as Paleolithic diet, autoimmune diet, GAPS diet, Okinawa diet, food guide according to the study of China, Mediterranean diet, intermittent fasting, ketogenic diet, detox diet, Montignac diet, diet Dunkan, Atkins diet, macrobiotic diet, vegetarian diet, vegan diet, and so on.

Some of the diets are supported by the official scientific community, and others are not. However, from my point of view and experience, all are valid depending on each person, moment, and circumstance. In addition, we all have much to discover, including the official scientific community.

All diets or eating guides have something in common, which is to restrict food to improve digestion. And by improving digestion, more nutrients are obtained with less effort. The function of our digestive system is optimized, and health is improved.

On the planet, energy is neither created nor destroyed; it simply transforms. And our digestive system transforms the energy of food into useful energy for our body.

Consuming less quantity, as long as it allows us to reach the energy we need, means being more sustainable with the environment and with our body. Our body becomes more efficient in all its functions and stays healthier and younger. And the same goes for the planet. But how do you get to eat a small amount, feel satiated, be nourished, and have energy?

Success is based on the perfect combination and processing of food. That is, to balance macronutrients and boost micronutrients. The components of the food and drink we consume interact with each other.

Knowing how to process and combine them correctly, we improve digestion and maximize their bioavailability. This will bring us enormous benefits for our health (better nutrition) and for the planet (better use of resources). An example is as follows:

Kale, strawberries, corn, eggs, black garlic, and olive oil. Balance the macronutrients of each meal. For example, according to the healthy dish of the example, for an adult: 2 boiled eggs (animal protein has greater bioavailability), 200gr. Sweet corn (carbohydrates: starch and sugar), 100gr. Of kale (curly cabbage) massaged with olive oil (healthy fats) and strawberries (vitamins, minerals, and fiber).

Combine micronutrients to improve digestion and enhance its nutritional value—for example, green leafy vegetables with healthy fats. Green leafy vegetables help digest fats, and fats help absorb vitamins from vegetables.

Save work for the intestine, eating predigested food, for example: crushed, marinated, massaged, fermented vegetables; yogurt; dextrinized bread; hot proteins; natural sweet food.

Distinguish between physiological and emotional hunger. And eat only in the presence of the first.

Not as a Perfect Meal

Dietary models are endlessly followed by dietary rules, good and bad food, restrictions, exclusions. But in reality, nutrition is not a complete science. Of course, you generally know what you need to be in shape and healthy, but that is not an immortal guarantee. You can't get sick. Worrying about the finer details of the diet and surprising all the small nutrients is unlikely to actually be healthy because excessive concentration on nutrition causes anxiety and appetite.

Food concerns can even have negative physiological consequences. For me, the best meal means having a healthy balance of food, and a healthy relationship with food, flexible—no strict rules or restrictions.

Dealing With Leftovers

Portion sizes being served in restaurants have increased over time, and even if they hadn't, it's unlikely that a standardized serving in a restaurant will be the exact right amount of food for everyone who orders a particular dish. Everyone's appetite is different from day to day and meal to meal, so it's impossible that your order will perfectly meet your exact requirements. Applying your mindful-eating skills will help you find the amount of food that's appropriate for you.

Sometimes that means having leftovers. You can really struggle with this, especially because there's a big emphasis on reducing food waste. So here are some ideas for dealing with leftovers:

- Ask for any leftovers to be boxed up (take your own containers if you're super-organized)

- Eat them the next day

- Give them to your housemate, kid, or partner

- Offer them to a rough sleeper

- If you know a place has huge portions or you know you're not that hungry, consider sharing the dish (and maybe ordering a few sides to go along with it)

The Foundation of a Healthy Diet

I will show you the secret of a healthy meal, so I hope you will sit down. Are you ready? Because this may just blow off your socks! Balance and diversity.

Surely it may not be the most revolutionary advice ever: surely enough to drink green juice or "coffee gives cancer, waits, no, coffee cures cancer," and the media It's not as cool as afraid, but it's very solid advice. And chances are you are already nailing it, and if you are not, you are doing it better than you think.

- **Balance**: In nutrition, when we talk about balance, we mean that balance is achieved over time. Not all meals need to be perfectly balanced. It does not mean every day. Your body won't reset magically at midnight. Balance is achieved over days, weeks, and months. It is an average time, not a meal once a day. If you don't eat for five days a day, you won't be undernourished!

Too often, sensible meal advice is taken to the extreme. The public health message to pay attention to sugar intake has been distorted and altered to "sugar is toxic and must be cut off immediately." But we know that restrictions and deprivation are completely counterfeited and go too far, overeating and overeating these forbidden foods.

Moderation tends to cherish itself when paying attention to how food makes us feel and eat according to hunger, fullness, and satisfaction. We are drawn to balanced food. Because it feels good, stop feeling obsessed with the food on the previous shit list.

- **Diversity**: Restricted diets tend to be more restrictive. In other words, we don't always get the most diverse but prefer to stick to "safe" food. We will eat the same food over and over again. When we eat more intuitively and turn consciousness to what we are eating, it tends to get a lot of variety because it is satisfying and tasteful, but this is what makes us wider.

This also helps from a nutritional perspective, meaning a wide range of foods and nutrients to cover a wide range of nutrients.

Eating nutritious food should not sacrifice taste. Even if the nutrients are high, you don't need to eat that shit if you have food you can't really stand. Gentle nutrition is not deprivation or eating something you don't like.

Raw granola coated with spirulina is slightly higher in iron (or whatever it makes up) and does not need to be eaten. If you taste junk, do not eat. Think of a new creative way to enjoy vegetables and whole grains. I don't like quinoa. No problem.

There are almost endless combinations of other foods that will help you get enough fiber and protein. Don't like kale? Don't mess it up! Nutrition should not sacrifice food taste. There is no need to do so! This may seem natural, but you'll have to deprive yourself of delicious food during the day and hang around at night.

CHAPTER 19:

The Right Foods to Help Balance Your Body

The neat thing with our health is that we are able to balance our bodies and keep them as healthy as possible with the help of some of the foods that we eat. Often eating the wrong foods are the reason why we end up with a lot of problems in our health.

On the other hand, when we are able to change our diets around, we can make our health so much better. It is not always instant because our bodies have to take some time to heal and get better. But the more that we can eat good foods that are high in vitamins and nutrients, and healthy carbs and good protein, the better our whole bodies will be.

There are a lot of good foods that we are able to enjoy that will help us to feel better and can get us in the best health. But there are also a lot of foods that we need to avoid in order to make sure that we are not causing issues and making our blood sugars and insulin levels, or even our cholesterol levels, to go back up.

Some of the different foods that we should consider enjoying in order to keep our bodies healthy and can help to fuel our body and our minds in a healthy manner includes:

Fruits and Vegetables

First, we can talk about vegetables. There are a lot of vegetables out there that we are able to consume, and all of them are going to be good for increasing our health, filling us up with fewer calories, and so much more. It is best to go for a lot of variety when you pick out your vegetables. This helps you to get more nutrients out of your meals and makes sure that you are not going to get bored with what you are eating, either.

Then it is time to move on to the fruits that we want to eat. There are lots of yummy choices when it comes to the fruits that we want to eat as well. Things like bananas, strawberries, blueberries, grapes, apples, peaches, and more can be a wonderful addition to our diet plans. They have vitamins and nutrients and lots of great things inside. Plus, they are sweet, so that can help when you have some cravings for the old sugary products you used to enjoy.

There are a lot of diet plans out there that are going to talk about all of the healthy fruits and vegetables that you are able to eat, and it is best if you can get a lot of these into your diet as well. The more, the merrier, for the most part, as long as you stay within the calorie guidelines that you are meant to.

With some of the diets out there, though, like the low carb diet, you do need to be careful with the amount of these you eat. The good news is there are a lot of low carb fruits and vegetables that you are able to consume and can add to your diet, so as long as you are careful with some of the other options, you will be fine getting all of the nutrients that you need from these along the way.

The one thing to remember here when working with lots of healthy fruits and vegetables is that we need to focus on the variety of what you are eating. If you just consume the exact same fruits and the exact same vegetables all of the time, then you are going to end up with a lot of issues along the way. This is going to get boring really quickly, and it is likely that following this process is going to give you a lack of nutrients at some point.

Add a lot of color to the plate that you are using. The more colors that you are able to add to each plate, the better because this ensures that you are able to get a ton of nutrients without having to count it all out or worry about how this is going to work at all. Plus, it is one of the best ways to make sure that we are able to see some improvements in how much we enjoy the diet plan that we are on in the first place.

Healthy Grains

When it comes to your diet plan, focusing on some healthy grains can be a great way to get started as well. These are going to provide us with some of the energy that we need, without all the ups and downs that can happen to our bodies when we deal with the processed baked goods and white bread. You do not want to eat too many of these, or they can cause some problems with your health and having too many carbs. But having some of the good whole grains with our meals can be a good way to balance out our blood sugars and help us to feel better overall.

On the other hand, there are a lot of good and healthy grains that we are able to eat instead. These are going to have a lot of healthy nutrients inside of them, and they digest well so that it can keep us full and satisfied for a lot longer period of time as well. Go for the whole grain and the multigrain options, and you are sure to take care of your body and provide it with some of the nutrition and the other goodness that it needs.

Dairy Products

Now it is time for the calcium. Having lots of calcium in your diet is so important in helping you to stay healthy and happy. Eating healthy sources of protein, including milk, yogurts, cheeses, and more, can be a welcome addition to any diet plan that you are on. They give your body lots of protein, calcium, and even vitamin D that the body needs.

Protein Sources

When you are trying to balance out your body and make it feel better, adding in some higher quality protein sources can be so important. Protein is so good for balancing out our blood sugar levels and helping us to be as healthy as possible. And they are good at filling us up, helping our muscles to stay strong, and so much more. And if we are able to choose the right kinds of proteins that will help us to get other vitamins and minerals, you are able to stay even healthier as well.

Lots of fish and lean cuts of chicken and turkey are good for helping with this. Things like ham, bacon, and ground beef are not necessarily that bad, but they can have some higher levels of saturated fats, so we have to be careful with those. Having them on occasion is not going to hurt too much, so they can be sources to consider. But the leaner cuts, the chicken and turkey and fish, are often better choices to go with to help keep your body as healthy as possible.

Healthy Fats

One thing that a lot of people forget about when they are worried about their health and losing weight is to take on the right amount of healthy fats. You need to make sure that your diet includes some fats in the meals that you eat. There are differences between the healthy fats that help your body absorb the good vitamins and nutrients that you need and the bad fats that come in processed and fast foods that are so bad for your body.

There are several sources where we are able to get some of these healthy fats. Choices like whole milk, olive oil, and even fish can be great sources that also have some of the other vitamins and minerals that your body needs in order to stay as healthy as possible. Try to add in a few of these to your day and see how much more energy you have, without adding in too many calories or a bunch of bad things.

Foods to Avoid

First, processed and packaged foods need to be taken out. These may make life easier and can taste good, but they have a ton of sugars and carbs, and even sodium, along with other things that are going to cause some havoc in our bodies. It is best to avoid anything that is in the freezer section at the grocery store, along with fast foods and so much more.

We also need to be careful about the baked goods that we try to enjoy as well. It is fine to have these on occasion as a treat.

We need to cut out the baked goods, candy, and more so that we can just eat sugars that are all-natural, like what we find in fruits and vegetables, and avoid all of the ones that are bad for us.

Depending on the diet plan you choose to go on, it is possible that there will be a few other foods that you need to avoid as well. If you go on a low carb diet like the Ketogenic diet, for example, then you will want to limit a lot of the carbs that you are consuming. Then there are options that go the other way that ask you to cut down on the meats and animal products that you consume on a regular basis. And some are even lower in fats and will ask you to cut down on how many of those you are consuming as well.

And make sure to not drink a lot of fruit juices, pops and sodas, and energy drinks. These are going to be full of lots of sugars and caffeine that can mess with our bodies and can make us feel bad as well. Try to keep these as just occasional things that you have once in a while and not something that you should have on a daily basis.

CHAPTER 20:

Stopping Emotional Eating

Emotional eating occurs typically when your food becomes a tool that you use in responding to any internal or external emotional cues. It's normal for human beings to tend to react to any stressful situation and the painful feelings that they have. Whenever you have stressful emotions, you tend to run after a bag of chips or bars of chocolate, a large pizza, or a jar of ice cream to distract yourself from that emotional pain. The foods that you crave at that moment are referred to as comfort food. Those foods contain a high calorie or high carbohydrate with no nutritional value.

Do you know that your appetite increases whenever you are stressed, and whenever you're stressed, you tend to make poor eating habits? Stress is associated with weight gain and weight loss. You tend to cleave unto food when you are under intense pressure and intense emotions like boredom or sadness. Now that's emotion napping, and it is the way that your body relieves itself from the stress and gets the energy needed to overcome its over-dependence on food. Usually, get you to the point whereby you don't eat healthy anymore.

Emotional eating is a chronic issue that affects every gender, both male and female, but research have shown that women are more prone to emotional eating than men. Emotional eaters tend to incline towards salty, sweet, fatty, and generally high-calorie foods. Usually, these foods are not healthy for the body, and even if you choose to eat them, you should only consume them in moderation. Emotional eating, especially indulging in unhealthy food, end up affecting your weight.

Emotional eating was defined as eating in response to intense, passionate emotions. Many studies reveal that having a positive mood can reduce your food intake, so you need to start accepting the fact that positive emotions are now part of emotional eating in the same way that negative emotions are part of emotional eating.

Effects of Emotional Eating

So here are some effects of emotional eating.

Intense Nausea

When you are food binging, the food provides a short-term distraction to the emotions that you are facing, and more than often, you will tend to eat very quickly, and as a result, you will overeat. This will then result in stomach pains or nausea, which can last for one or two days. So, it is essential to concentrate on the problem that is causing you to stress instead of eating food to solve that problem.

Feeling Guilty

The next one is feeling guilty. Occasionally, you may use food as a reward to celebrate something that is not necessarily bad. It is essential to celebrate the little wings that you have in life, and if food is the way you choose to celebrate it, then you should want to eat healthy meals instead of going for unhealthy snacks. However, when food becomes your primary mechanism for coping with emotional stress whenever you feel stressed, upset, lonely, angry, or exhausted, then you will open the fridge and find yourself in an unhealthy cycle, without even being able to target the root cause of the problem that is making you stressed. Furthermore, you will be filled with guilt. Even after all the emotional damage has passed away, you will still be filled with remorse for what you have done and for the unhealthy lifestyle that you choose to make at that moment, which will then lower your self-esteem. And then, you will go into another emotional eating outburst.

Weight-Related Health Issues

The next one is weight-related health issues. I'm sure that you are aware of how unhealthy eating affects your weight. Many researchers have discovered that emotional eating affects weight, both positively and negatively. Generally, the foods that you crave during those emotional moments are high in sugar and high in salt and saturated fats. And in those emotional moments, you tend to eat anything that you can lay your hands on.

Now even though some healthy fast foods are available, many of them are still filled with salt, sugar, and trans-fat content. High carbohydrate food increases the demand for insulin in the body, which then promotes hunger more and more, and therefore you tend to eat more calories than you are supposed to consume. Consuming a high level of fat can have an immediate impact on your blood vessels, and it does that in the short-term. If you drink too much fat, your blood pressure will increase, and you will become hospitable to heart attack, kidney disease, and another cardiovascular disease. Many manufactured fats are created during food processing, and those fat are found in pizza, dough, crackers, fried pies, cookies, and pastries.

Do not be misinformed; no amount of saturated fat is healthy. If you continue to eat this kind of food, you'll be putting yourself at the risk of HDL and LDL, which is the right kind of cholesterol and the wrong kind of cholesterol. And to be frank, both of them will put your heart at risk of diabetes, high blood pressure, high cholesterol, obesity, and insulin resistance. So, these are some of the challenges that you will face when you engage in emotional eating outbursts.

How to Stop Emotional Eating Using Meditation

You already know what to eat, and you already know what is not to eat, and you already know what is right for your body and what is not suitable for your body. Even if you're not a nutritionist or a health coach or a fitness activist, you already know these things. But when you are alone, you tend to engage in emotional eating, and you successfully keep it to yourself and make sure that no one knows about it. It is just like you surrender your control for food to a food demon, and when that demon possesses you, you become angry, sad, and stress at once, and before you know what is happening, you have gone to your fridge, opened it, and begin to consume whatever is there.

As strong as you, once this food demon has possessed you, it will convince you that food is the only way to get out of that emotional turmoil that you are facing. So, before you know what is happening, you are invading your refrigerator and consuming that jar of almond butter that you promised yourself not to drink. And just a few seconds, you open the jar of almond butter, take the bottle, put it in your mouth, and close the door again. And you do it again and again and again, and before you know what is happening, you have leveled the jar up to halfway, and not a dent has been made on the initial in motion that you were eating over.

Now before you know it, if your consciousness catches up with you. You start to feel sad, guilt, and shame. The almond butter that you were eating didn't help you that much, not in the way that you wanted it to help you. So, if there is anything you need to realize, you now feel worse than you were one hour ago. And so, you make a promise that you won't repeat this again and that this is the last time that this will happen.

You promised yourself never to share an entrance with that almond butter again, but then you realize that this is what you have been doing to the gluten-free cookies, to that ice cream, and hot chocolate before now. If this is your behavior, then you'll be able to relate to this. Emotional eating is a healthy addition that you must stop. It is more of a habit and one not easy to control. So, there is hope for you if you are engaging in emotional eating today. You have to be able to have control over yourself and over your emotional eating. There are many strategies that you can use to combat emotional eating, and one of them is meditation.

Now when it comes to emotional eating and weight management, it is essential to acknowledge the connection between our minds and our bodies. Today we live in a hectic and packed world that is weighing us down. However, mindful meditation can be a powerful tool to help you to be able to create a rational relationship with the food that you eat. One of the essential things about overcoming emotional eating is not to avoid the emotions, but rather to face them head-on and accept them the way they are and agree that they are a crucial part of your life.

If you want to put a stop to emotional eating, then you need to be able to shift your beliefs and worthiness. You need to be able to create a means to cope with unhealthy situations. It is essential to note that meditation will not cure your emotional eating completely. Instead, it will help you to examine and rationalize all the underlining sensations that are leading to emotional eating in your life. For emotional eaters, the feeling of guilt, shame, and low self-esteem are widespread.

Frequently these negative create judgment in their mind and triggers unhealthy eating patterns, and they end up feeling like an endless self-perpetuating loop. Meditation helps you to be able to develop a non-judgmental mindset about observing your reality. And that mindset will be able to help with you and suppress your emotions negative feelings, without even trying to suppress them or comfort them with foods.

Develop the Mind and Body Connection

Meditation will help you to develop the mind and body connection. And once you're able to create that connection, you will be able to distinguish between emotional eating and physical hunger. Once you can differentiate between that, you'll be able to recognize your cues for hunger and safety. You will instantly tell when your desire is not related to physical hunger. Research indicates that medication will help to strengthen your prefrontal cortex, which is the part of the brain that helps you with will power. That part of the brain is responsible for allowing us to resist the impulse is within us. Mindfulness will help the calls to eat even when they're not hungry.

By strengthening that prefrontal cortex, you'll be able to get comfortable at observing those impulses without acting on them. If you want to get rid of the unhealthy habit and start to build new ones, you need to be able to work on your prefrontal cortex, and you can only do that with meditation. Once you start meditating, you will begin reaping the benefits. You will learn how to be able to live more in the present. You'll become more aware of your thinking patterns, and in no time, you will be able to become conscious of how you treat food. You'll be able to make the right choice when it comes to food.

CHAPTER 21:

Daily Weight Loss Motivation

Before you can begin using mind exercises and meditations to do things such as help you burn fat, you need to make sure that you set yourself up properly for your meditation sessions. Each meditation will consist of you entering a deep state of relaxation, following guided hypnosis, and then awakening yourself out of this state of relaxation. If done properly, you will find yourself experiencing the stages of changed mindset and changed behavior that follows the session.

These exercises will involve a visualization practice; however, if you find that visualization is generally difficult for you, you can simply listen. The key here is to ensure that you keep as open of a mind as possible so that you can stay receptive to the information coming through these guided meditations.

Mind Exercises to Find Your Motivation

Start by gently closing your eyes and drawing your attention to your breath. As you do, I want you to track the next five breaths, gently and intentionally lengthening them to help you relax as deeply as you can. With each breath, breathe into the count of five and out to the count of seven. Starting with your next breath in, Count 1-10.

Start repeatedly counting from 1-5. Do this three times while inhaling and exhaling.

Now that you are starting to feel relaxed, I want you to draw your awareness into your body. First, become aware of your feet. Feel your feet deeply relaxing as you visualize any stress or worry melting away from your feet. Now, become aware of your legs. Feel any stress or worry melting away from your legs as they begin to relax completely. Next, become aware of your glutes and pelvis, allowing any stress or worry to fade away as they completely relax simply. Now, become aware of your entire torso, allowing any stress or worry to melt away from your torso as it relaxes completely. Next, become aware of your shoulders, arms, hands, and fingers. Allow the stress and worry to melt away from your shoulders, arms, hands, and fingers as they relax completely. Now, let the stress and worry melt away from your neck, head, and face. Feel your neck, head, and face relaxing as any stress or worry melts away completely.

As you deepen into this state of relaxation, I want you to take a moment to visualize the space in front of you. Imagine that in front of you, you are standing there looking back at yourself. See every inch of your body as it is right now standing before you, casually, as you simply observe yourself. While you do, see what parts of your body you want to reduce fat so that you can create a healthier, stronger body for yourself. Visualize the fat in these areas of your body, slowly fading away as you begin to carve out a healthier, leaner, and stronger body underneath. Notice how effortlessly this extra fat melts away as you continue to visualize yourself becoming a healthier and more vivacious version of yourself.

Now, I want you to visualize what this healthier, leaner version of yourself would be doing. Visualize yourself going through your typical daily routine, except the perspective of your healthier self. What would you be eating? When and how would you be exercising? What would you spend your time doing? How do you feel about yourself? How different do you feel when you interact with the people around you, such as your family and your co-workers? What does life feel like when you are a healthier, leaner version of yourself?

Spend several minutes visualizing how different your life is now that your fat has melted away. Feel how natural it is for you to enjoy these healthier foods and how easy it is to moderate your cravings and indulgences when you choose to treat yourself. Notice how easy it is for you to engage in exercise and how exercise feels enjoyable and like a wonderful hobby, rather than a chore that you must force yourself to commit to every day. Feel yourself genuinely enjoying life far more, all because the unhealthy fats that weigh you down and disrupt your health have faded away. Notice how easy it was for you to get here and how easy it is for you to continue to maintain your health and wellness as you continue to choose better and better choices for you and your body.

Feel how much you respect your body when you make these healthier choices and how much you genuinely care about yourself. Notice how each meal and exercise feels like an act of self-care rather than a chore you are forcing yourself to engage in. Feel how good it feels to do something for you—for your wellbeing. When you are ready, take that visualization of yourself and send the image out far, watching it become nothing more than a spec in your field of awareness. Then, send it out into the ether, trusting that your subconscious mind will hold onto this vision of yourself and work daily on bringing this version of you into your current reality.

Now, awaken back into your body where you sit right now. Feel yourself feeling more motivated, more energized, and more excited about engaging in the activities that will improve your health and help you burn your fat. As you prepare to go about your day, hold onto that visualization and those feelings that you had of yourself, and trust that you can have this wonderful experience in your life. You can do it!

Daily Weight Loss Motivation With Mini Habits

Once you have set your plans, written your affirmations, chosen your mantras, begun to practice all the meditation and mindfulness techniques you have learned, what is next? Like anything that you have invested in, it is important to perform maintenance. Being able to reach and stay at your goal weight is only part of the picture because what you are working on is a total lifestyle change. You want your habits and your decision-making to match the life you want to be living. Let us recap the methods you have learned and show you how to apply them to the future of your new self.

Making Habits Count

We spent a lot of time thinking about the importance of habits. It can be hard to see the behavioral patterns in our lives until we try to change them. By making a conscious decision to take something that is not conducive to weight loss and replacing it with a habit, you have already taken a step towards improvement. It is said that no one can change unless they want to change, and that is very true.

Habits are the key that can tie all of your other efforts together. You can make a habit of reading your affirmations and reciting your mantras. You can replace a television or video game habit with exercise and meditation. You can break the habit of eating convenience foods by mindfully making a shopping list. Everything we have talked about in this entire book can be tied back into making, breaking, or replacing a habit.

Positive Words for a Positive Outcome

Here is just one last reminder to think positive! We talked a lot about the power of positivity and how it can impact everything you do. Words do have a tremendous amount of power, which is why mantras can be so vital to reaching a weight loss goal.

When you learn to apply mantras to your goals, you are assigning power to positive words, and when you shun the negativity of others, you are taking power away from their words. Do not let your life be a power struggle. Use strong, upbeat words to describe yourself. Be sure that if a sentence contains both negative and positive statements, that you phrase your words to frame and emphasize the positive component.

It can be difficult to change your mindset, and it will take work. But do not get discouraged, and do not allow negativity to rent any space in your brain. Every day is a new day to wake up and commit to positivity. Think carefully about your words and mind how you speak to and about yourself. By making a conscious effort to be positive, you will have a great day and another until being positive becomes your new way of life.

Taking Time for Meditation and Mindfulness

You may be wondering how you will make time for all this positivity, habit formation, and affirmation reading. Now we are going to add meditation and mindfulness to the mix. We do only have so many hours in the day, but all these elements are so crucial to reaching your goals. So how can you do it? How do you find the time to stick to your plan?

The answer is you make time. When you commit to change yourself, there will be sacrifices. You can try getting up a half-hour early or carving out time after work. If you have a support system around you, ask someone to watch your kids while you go to the gym or take them off the school bus to have a few extra minutes to yourself in the afternoon. Where there is a will—and you have the will—there is always a way.

You can combine your affirmation and meditation time into your wake up and bedtime routines—practice mindfulness in the shower. Recite mantras during your grocery shop. You can, and you will find the time. Yes, things like yoga and visualization can be a little time consuming, but the more you practice all your techniques, the more efficient you will become. Be creative about how you spend your time. If you need to make yourself a loose schedule of when you are going to practice your self-hypnosis methods, it will help you stay on track.

Tying It All Together

You have probably decided what methods you would like to use to aid you on your weight-loss journey. Any of the techniques outlined in this book will be useful tools for you as you move forward. But what happens once you reached your initial goal? You do not want to slip back into your bad habits or let go of the positivity you have injected into your life.

You will also probably be fighting the urge to weigh yourself frequently. Do not give in to this temptation. While it is important to monitor yourself, it is never a good idea to obsess over the scale. You want to continue to keep a positive self-image based on how you feel about yourself and not about a number. If you are concerned that you may gain back some weight, continue to weigh yourself once a week and adjust your regimen accordingly. Being able to self-adjust based on your current circumstance is a sign of success. You have done all the hard work; now, it is time to use what you have learned to keep your weight in check.

CHAPTER 22:

Daily Weight Loss Meditation

Meditation is in fashion. As soon as you tell someone that you have a problem, it is a rare occasion when they do not recommend you practice it. It does not matter if the problem is mental or physical.

Sometimes, people's insistence leads us to reject a plan idea. However, would it not be more interesting to ask why so many people agree to advise you the same thing? Interest in Eastern cultures brought the influence of ideas to the forefront. And they are our existence's nucleus. Nutrition and physical exercise promote our body's optimal working. Yet, it is also true that when our emotions aren't controlled, the brain secretes substances that affect our body and mind. Therefore, physical sufferings or thoughts that make life difficult for us can appear. In this way, meditation helps to keep us safe.

Meditation lowered inflammation levels. Beyond what happened in mind, they find an inflammation measure lower than before the investigation. It indicates that perception benefits go beyond what would appear.

The group manager warns, however, that the exact extent of its benefits cannot yet be defined. Nevertheless, the observation is adequate to multiply scientists' efforts in this regard. It is no longer about Buddhist experiences or self-help customers who can't control. We have evidence. However, intentional meditation enhances our quality of life. In addition, the fact that its effects last four months means that it is a long-term practice that benefits us. Given the number of harmful elements to which we are exposed without being able to do anything, it seems reasonable to bet on this option.

All this shows us how the first step to improving our health is to listen to our bodies.

It is very unlikely that the effects you notice when introducing a new habit constitute a mere imagination. Therefore, from here, we want to thank the efforts of many people who have defended an alternative lifestyle—another class of medicine.

Even when they have been treated as "enlightened" and a little sane, their constancy and the defense of their values have been translated into a scientific study that has proved them right and from which we will all benefit.

Practicing Anti-Stress Meditation at Home

We know that sometimes it costs. How to combine our daily obligations with that moment of anti-stress meditation? We get up with things to do and arrive at bed with a mind full of those tasks and commitments that must be fulfilled for the following day.

Be careful if the preceding paragraph is an example of what you always live in your day today. It is essential that you know how to organize times and set limits, control all those pressures that do not allow you to get rest.

Ideally, you learn to balance your life. Where you are always the priority of taking care of your health and your emotions, stress can hurt you a lot, and you should see it as an enemy to dominate, to do small to be able to handle it properly. We explain how to practice anti-stress meditation.

1. Emotional Agenda

Do you keep an agenda in your day to day of the things you should do? Of your obligations, appointments, meetings, appointments with teachers of children, or your visit to the doctor?

Do the same with your emotions, with your personal needs. Spend at least one hour or two hours for yourself each day. To do what you like, to be alone, and to practice anti-stress meditation. Your emotions have priority; make a hole in your day today. You deserve it, and you need it.

2. A moment of Tranquility

It doesn't matter where it is. In your room, in the kitchen or in a park. You must be calm and surrounded by an environment that is pleasant, placid, and comforting. If you want, put on the music that you like, but you must be alone.

3. Regulate Your Breathing

Let's now take care of our breathing. Once you are comfortable, start to take a deep breath through your nose. Allow your chest to swell, then let this air out little by little through your mouth. If you repeat it six or seven times, you will begin to notice a comforting tingling through your body, and you feel better and calmer.

4. Focus Thoughts

What will we do after? Visualize those pressures that concern you most. Are you pressured at work? Do you have problems with your partner? Visualize those images and keep breathing. The tension should soften, the nerves should lose their intensity, and the fear will soften. You will feel better little by little.

5. Positive Images

Once you have focused on those images, what more pressure they cause on your being? Let's now go on to visualize pleasant things, aspects that you would like to be living, and that would make you happy.

They must be simple things: a walk on the beach, you touching the bark of a tree, you walk through a quiet city where the sun illuminates your face and where the rumor of nearby coffee shops envelops you with a pleasant smell of coffee. Easy things make you happy. Visualize it and keep breathing deeply.

6. The Silence

Now we close our eyes. At least for two minutes. Try not to think about anything; just let the silence envelop you. You are at peace, and you are well. There is no pressure. There are only you and a quiet world where there are no pressures and threats, and everything is warm and pleasant.

7. Open Your Eyes in a Renewed Way

It is time to open your eyes and breathe normally again. Look around without moving, without getting up. Don't do it, or you'll run the risk of getting dizzy. Allow about five minutes to pass before you walk again. Surely you feel much better, lighter, and without any pressure on your body.

8. New Perspectives

Now that you feel more relaxed try to think about what you can do to find yourself better day by day. Being a little happier sometimes requires that we have to make small changes. And the good thing about anti-stress meditation is that it is slowly changing us inside.

It requires us to make small changes to find the balance so that the body and the mind feel in tune again, and the pressures, the anxieties go out of our body like the smoke that escapes through a window.

Simple Meditation Exercises

Stress accumulates like oil. Paradoxically, as one increases, the other declines. Therefore, stress and energy can fuel a wide variety of sources. For example, stress may feed on problems in various places or simply a life pattern marked by a lack of breaks. We will present simple meditation exercises to help relieve this stress.

Indeed, meditation encourages self-awareness. It is an ancient Indian peculiar millennial technique, popular in Buddhist and Hindu beliefs. It's become common in the West in recent years.

One of the advantages of meditation is an increase in the ability to focus, which is the starting point for many other advantages, such as better memory. This also usually enables physical and emotional relaxation. This may also improve our immune system against threats to our safety.

Without further explanation, let's add a set of basic meditation exercises that we can put into action to optimize its benefits.

1. Focus Your Attention on Breathing

The first of the simple meditation exercises is also one of the easiest to incorporate into our routine. We will do it more easily if we can adopt a relaxed position with semi-open eyes.

It is also good to focus on our breathing without trying to vary the parameters. It's about perceiving the air coming in and going out. At this moment, it is common to be distracted by different thoughts. Our mission will be to ignore them until they lose their strength.

2. Countdown

This technique is extremely simple and is of great use when it comes to meditating. With your eyes closed, count back from high numbers such as 50 or 100 until you reach zero. The goal of this practice is to focus our attention on a single thought/activity. In this way, we will be able to eliminate the sensations produced by the rest of the stimulations.

3. Scan Our Own Body

This is the most interesting one of many and simple meditation exercises. We only need to reassess the different parts of our body. For this, it is recommended to place ourselves in a place of weak stimulation. Then we will focus our attention on all parts of our body, starting from the head to finish with the feet.

We can contract and release the different muscle groups to become aware of their presence and their movement. It is a rather attractive way to observe ourselves and to perceive in detail the sensations of our body.

4. Observe Dynamically

This exercise is focused on studying our climate. Let's start with a comfortable position; the best is sitting with your eyes closed. We'll then open them to close them for a moment. Before that, we'll have to focus on what's learned.

We'll be able to think about the various sensations that we're generating the stimulations that came to us. We may list them; think of each object's shapes and colors, or name. Furthermore, if we know this at home, it might be a good way to experience our home differently.

5. Meditating in Motion

Another basic meditation exercise we can put into action is based on our body's feedback of fun stimuli as it moves. For this, interaction with nature is recommended.

For example, we can take a few steps on the beach or in the woods and enjoy the warmth of the sun on our faces, the wind caresses, or the touch of plants and water on our hands. It can also be another way to make a personal observation, thinking about our body's movements as we walk.

6. Meditate With Fire

Finally, we can use fire as a symbolic purification item to focus our meditation. We may concentrate on a campfire in nature or something simpler: a candle's flame. It will allow us to experience the heat sensations associated with fire and the shadows reflecting on the surrounding objects.

On the other side, we can list and burn negative items in our everyday lives. This positive gesture that can be performed symbolically or factually helps us free ourselves from our worries of something we have no influence over.

CHAPTER 23:

Daily Weight Loss Affirmations

Affirmations are verbal statements that help us to affirm something we believe. So often, we say negative affirmations to ourselves without even realizing it. Recognize those negative thoughts and replace them with the positive statements that we have listed below. Repeat these to yourself daily. Write them down on a piece of paper or have notes on them that you leave throughout your house. Remember to practice your breathing exercises that we have learned through the other mindset exercises and keep an open mind as always.

Affirmations to Lose Weight Naturally

Losing weight is more than just looking good to me. I understand that I need to live a healthy lifestyle to feel better all of the time.

I know how to lose weight, and actually, I choose to do this naturally because it helps me be healthier. I know what I need to do to get the things I deserve from this life.

I am capable of reaching all of the goals that I set for myself, and I am the one who decides what I do next with my life.

I recognize that it's essential for me to be patient throughout this process. I can wait for the results because I know that I will get everything that I want in the end. I do not punish myself because I don't achieve a goal as fast as I had hoped initially. I nourish myself throughout this process. I continuously look for ways to encourage myself and build my self-esteem because I know that is what is going to help me feel the best in the end. I can control my impulses. I know how not to act on my highest urges. I recognize the methods that will help me to enable myself to work harder in the end. I am happy because I know how to say no.

I can turn away when I'm confronted with an impulse. I am more durable than the biggest cravings that I have. I am proud of my ability to have a high level of willpower. I trust myself around certain foods and recognize that what tempts me does not control me.

I look at the things that I already have in my life instead of only paying attention to something that I don't have.

This is the way that will help me better achieve everything that I desire. I do not allow distractions to keep me from getting the things that I want. I can stay focused on my goals so that I can create the life that I deserve. In the end, even when I am tempted by something or somebody else, I know how to push through this urge and instead focus on my goals. I will wait for everything. Love is coming to me because I know that, when it does, I will feel entirely fulfilled. I am enjoying the journey and the process that it takes to get the body that I want. I recognize that small milestones are worth celebrating.

I do not wait for one big goal to be reached to be happy with myself. I look for all the methods needed to achieve greatness in this life. I understand that a temporary desire to eat something unhealthy is not worth giving up on all of my goals. I know how to distract myself from my biggest cravings so that I can do something healthy instead. I recognize that doing something small is better than doing nothing at all. Even on the days that I don't want to go to the gym, I do something at home to work out so that I can at least accomplish something minor.

Just getting started is the hardest part for me, but I know how to work through those feelings now. I am emotionally aware of what might be holding me back so that I don't allow myself to be tempted by distractions.

I control my feelings and my urges so that I don't do anything that I regret. I am happy because I am knowledgeable about the things that make me who I am.

I forgive myself when I do act on an impulse. I don't punish myself or deprive my body of the first things that it needs just because I did something wrong. I sacrifice certain things that I want but never to a point where I cause punishment or torture on myself. I am successful because I am dedicated. I have strong willpower because I am successful. I move through my life with gratitude and always look to appreciate the things that I have around me. I can pick myself up when I'm feeling weak.

I am appreciative of even the hard parts of my life because they create the person that I am. I am a talented and influential person. I have control over my body, and nobody else does. I recognize my weaknesses, but in the same breath, I am very aware of my strengths. I balance my life with these things. I empower my strengths and thrive when I am in an environment that helps me grow. I recognize my weaknesses, and I always look for ways to turn them around to live more happily and healthily after. I cook meals for myself because it makes me feel healthier and more reliable in the end.

I am going to get the dream body that I want because I can recognize things that might be healthy or unhealthy for me. I move my body at least once a day. I always feel better after I agree to a workout rather than if I try to avoid one. I can give myself rest when I need it. I don't push myself when I'm too stressed out because I know that this isn't going to help me get the things that I want.

I can always find motivation and passion within myself. I set my own goals, and I set newer and bigger ones after I achieved ones that I already completed. I do not procrastinate with my goals. I know what I have to do every single day to reach these goals, and I always look for ways to go above and beyond as well. I am continually improving the methods that I use to live a healthy lifestyle. I self-reflect so that I can find real solutions to any issues that I might face. I don't let what other people think to take over how I see myself. I am not afraid of judgment from other people because I know that not everything negative that somebody thinks about me is right.

I make the right decision for my body. I understand that even if I make wrong decisions, sometimes, they all play a vital role in making me the person that I am today. These struggles are something that I had to undergo to become the powerful individual that I am.

I am continually losing weight because of all this dedication and passion. I feel lighter, happier, and healthier. I am free. I am pure and clean. I am collected and calm. I am peaceful, and I am so glad. I heal myself through my weight loss. I take everything wrong that I did to my body in the past and turn it into something useful, as I exercise and make healthy choices. I am always getting closer and closer to the things that I want. I'm focused on pushing through my most significant setbacks to achieve the things that I deserve. I do not sit around and fantasize about what I want anymore. Instead, I know exactly how to get this. I believe in myself because I know that this is going to be an essential part of my journey. I trust my ability actually to lose weight, and I'm not afraid of what will happen if I don't. I know how to say these affirmations to myself when I feel better.

Other people like being around me. Others recognize my hard work. Others know that I deserve to have good things in my life. When I listened to my body, I can thrive. I recognize the things that my body tells me to get the best results possible.

I feel good, and I look even better. I look great, and I look incredible because of this. Not only does losing weight help my body to look better, but it also helps my soul, and that is something that can show through so quickly to other people. I choose to do things that are good for my body. I value myself, and I have virtue in all that I do. I add value to other people's lives, as well. I motivate myself, and therefore, I know how to motivate other people.

I am not afraid of anything. The worst thing that can happen to me is that I stop believing in myself. I will always be my best friend. I will still know how to encourage myself and include confidence in everything that I do. I love myself, and I am proud of the body that I have. I am perfect the way that I am, and I am beautiful. I am happy I am healthy, and I am free. I am focused, I am centered, and I am peaceful. I am stress-free and thankful. I have gratitude and love. I am attractive, and I am perfect. There is nothing that I need to punish myself for.

CHAPTER 24:

Daily Meditation for Self Esteem

So, you must talk about yourself with positive beliefs, even if you don't believe them at the time—fake it until you make it (as is the current phrase!) and in the case of weight problems, think like a slim person. A friend of mine who had put on a lot of weight said that she was surprised when she saw a picture of herself at that time, as she believed she was still slim—so it does work both ways!

Most people who are overweight are normally very critical and always speak negatively about themselves. They normally suffer from low self-worth and low self-esteem. The result is that, by doing this, they are perpetuating the problem. When you are speaking negatively to yourself, ask yourself if you would speak to a friend like that. The answer most probably will be that you wouldn't, so why on earth are you speaking like that to yourself? Stop it now!

You need to change your chatter from negative to positive even if you don't believe what you are saying. I hear you cry, "How can I be positive when I am fat?" but it is very important in the re-programming of your subconscious and your cells. Positive affirmations are an excellent way of re-programming, and these can be combined with EFTTM for stronger and quicker results.

Change "I am fat" to 'I am getting slimmer every day."

Change "I never lose weight" to "It gets easier every day to lose weight."

Changing Beliefs

People ask how they can change their beliefs, and luckily these days, there is a variety of techniques and therapies to help do this, but you also have to be careful not to fall back into any bad habits.

This relates to all areas in your life and not just to weight, so let me tell you a couple of stories:

I love Sunday nights as this is my pamper night where I have a long bath, face mask, and do my nails. Some of my friends hate Sunday night because they have to go back to work on Monday and they don't like their jobs. I have changed my perception of Sunday night so that I enjoy it, unlike my friends who dread it.

When I was made redundant, I opened up my own beauty salon, thinking that this was the best job in the world and something that I had always wanted to do. In reality, it was long hours for very little money, putting up with bolshie people who treated my staff and me appallingly. This taught me to love whatever job I was doing because there is no magic job that you will love for eight hours a day—each one has its ups and downs. Therefore, I changed my perception.

Other Therapies

Other therapies and techniques that are good for working on and changing the belief system are:

- EFTTM

- Affirmations/Afformations

- Hypnosis and Self Hypnosis

- NLP

Accepting Who You Are and Loving Yourself

If you despise your body, you get into a downward spiral of low self-esteem and self-loathing. You need to accept how you are now and be happy—remember that losing weight doesn't necessarily mean you are going to be any happier than you are now. Acceptance is also surrendering, and you give up the fight—once you have done this, you will find your angels and guides can give you more help.

Love your body and thank it for all it is doing for you at this moment. Your body is doing an excellent job, and it needs to be appreciated and thanked. You have to start changing your perception of yourself, and I know only too well that this is not easy.

Start loving yourself. This is not an ego love but a self-worth love, and you are worthy. For some unknown reason, it is very difficult to look at yourself in the mirror and say, "I love you," but this is important. Everybody has their unique traits, so write down yours and repeat them several times a day. If you don't love yourself and keep putting yourself down, you are opening up the path for everybody to treat you the same way.

EFTTM always incorporates "I love and accept myself." Sometimes people find this difficult to say, but after using EFTTM for a while, you realize that you are wonderful and that you love and respect yourself.

Canceling Negative Statements

Remember, if you say something negative, immediately say "CANCEL THAT LAST STATEMENT" —you can say it out loud (if you have made that comment) or under your breath if someone else has made a negative statement. If it helps, wear an elastic band around your wrist and ping it every time you make a negative statement—it stings and really stops you! It is very important to remember this technique as very often we say things all the time, which are a habit, such as "I am sorry."

If you want to apologize, say "I apologize" as this has a very different energy to, I am sorry.

These are positive statements to say after canceling a negative statement:

"I am healthy and well-nourished."

"I love myself, I love my body, and my excess fat disappears. "

"I am my ideal weight."

"I enjoy exercising several times a week."

"I can say "no.""

"My body is nourished."

"I am proud of my body."

"My metabolism works at 100%."

"I am spiritually, emotionally, and physically balanced."

Affirmations and Afformations

In personal development, an affirmation is a form of autosuggestion in which a statement of a desirable intention is repeated in order to implant it in our mind. An afformation is the same, but it is asked as a question because the subconscious loves questions and finds ways to answer them.

Louise Hay, who wrote You can heal your life, advocates affirmations for every area in life from health to work to home. Louise Hay believes that we cause our illnesses, and with the use of affirmations, we can begin the self-healing process.

Louise Hay's explanation for Bell's palsy is "total unspoken rage." When I was aged 20, my parents were moving house and insisted that I went with them. I tried very hard to refuse but was soon cowed by my mother, who insisted that I would be "out on the streets" if I didn't move with them. The morning of the move, I woke up with severe Bell's palsy. I ended up having an operation that involved shaving off most of my hair and cutting off my ear in order for the surgeon to scrape the nerve, causing the palsy. This, in fact, put me more into the clutches of my mother as I had an incredibly crooked face for two years and no hair! When I read "total unspoken rage," I knew that was exactly how I felt. From that moment on, I realized that we did cause our own illnesses; we just had to realize it.

I think everyone needs a copy of Louise Hay's books for reference as she talks about how to phrase the affirmations and how often to repeat them. You must always repeat an affirmation at least three times at once, and this set must then be repeated several times during the day. Remember, it is REPETITION that you need but do not include more than three positives in one statement. When I was doing a replacement, I wanted to put:

"I am beautiful, slim, fit, healthy, wealthy, and successful."

But with my teacher, we changed it to:

"I am slim, healthy, and fit."

The subconscious also strips out the word NOT, so it should never be in an affirmation statement. Using the example above, "I am not hungry" becomes "I am hungry"—another reason for weight gain.

If you give yourself a negative message, do the following:

- Stop and ping your elastic band.

- Say CANCEL that last statement immediately

- Immediately repeat a positive affirmation three times

Affirmations should be in your own words and must feel real to you to work properly. You need to say them out loud in a strong voice and really feel them and mean them. Here are a few examples of affirmations that you could use—if you wish to use an affirmation, just say it as a question, for example, 'Why am I so healthy?'

If you feel you are going to cheat:

"I'm losing weight now."

"I love the feeling of making progress."

To keep you on the straight and narrow:

"I'm getting fitter every day."

"I am feeling thinner today."

"I am getting slimmer and slimmer every day."

"I'm losing weight now."

"I am going to fit into the next size smaller any minute."

"I enjoy being healthy."

"My body is getting stronger, slimmer, and healthier every day."

"I feel so thin inside; my outer is just about to catch up."

"My metabolism is burning up all the food I eat."

"My weight will stay stable for the rest of my life."

"I am powerful."

Saying Affirmations Quickly

Recently a therapist told me of a brilliant way to get the most out of repeating your affirmations. If you are like me, you will have rakes of them, ranging from money to weight to career to health, and every time you repeat them, it becomes such a mouthful. So, type your affirmations up and give them a number. I then say, "Affirmation 1 will be XXXX," and then repeat this affirmation three times. This affirmation then becomes "Affirmation 1" or "1" in my subconscious.

In the future, instead of having to repeat all the affirmations say "Affirmation 1", "Affirmation 2," etc. They really roll off your tongue, and you can ensure that you get multiple repetitions done very quickly and efficiently!

Absorbing the Affirmations Quickly

As you are repeating your affirmation, tap around your scalp just outside and around your right ear (this is called temporal tapping). This helps absorb the affirmations into your brain more quickly than just saying them.

CHAPTER 25:

Meditations Techniques and Deep Sleep for Weight Loss

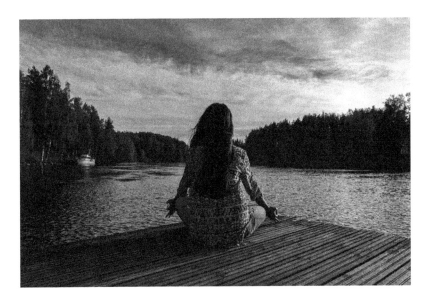

To properly set yourself up for a meditation experience, you need to make sure that you have a quiet space where you can engage in your meditation. You want to be as uninterrupted as possible so that you do not stir awake from your meditation session. In addition to having a quiet space, you should also ensure that your area is comfortable. For some of the meditations I will share, you can be lying down or doing this meditation before bed so that the information sinks in as you sleep. For others, you may want to stand upright, ideally with your legs crossed on the floor or with your feet on the floor when sitting in a chair. Staying in a sitting position, immensely during morning meditations, will help you stay awake and increase your motivation. Laying down during these meditations earlier in the day may result in you draining your energy and feeling exhausted completely rather than motivated. As a result, you may work against what you are trying to achieve.

The key here is to ensure that you keep as open a mind as possible to stay receptive to the information coming through these guided meditations.

Besides all of the above, listening to low music, using a pillow or a small blanket, and dressing in comfortable loose clothing will help you have better meditations. The more relaxed and comfortable you are, the more receptive you will be to your information within each meditation.

Fat Burning Meditation

This fat-burning meditation is a simple 30-minute meditation that will allow you to spend time visualizing your fat cells, reducing them into smaller and smaller cells until they practically vanish. By focusing on these hypnosis types, meditations help direct your subconscious mind to interact with your body to have a healthier and healthier body. When you intentionally draw your subconscious awareness into these activities, it encourages it to continue engaging in these activities on its own, even when you are not involved in your hypnosis session.

It is a great meditation to engage in during the day, anywhere from one to three times per week or at bedtime. They say that meditating right before you fall asleep can be incredibly potent, as you are contemplating during a time where your subconscious mind is extraordinarily active. Your conscious mind is already beginning to fall asleep. You are most likely to experience the relaxation and receptivity required for subconscious digestion and absorption during this time.

To begin this meditation, allow yourself to close your eyes and start to fade into a deep state of relaxation. Whenever I breathe, I relax more and more, noticing that I have fallen into a peaceful and lovely country. To help you deepen your vacation, I will guide you through a practice that will take you to the deepest level of peace possible. To do this, I want you to visualize yourself standing at the top of a set of stairs. As I count down from ten to one, I want you to imagine yourself walking down that flight of stairs, taking just one step at a time. With each step, you accept, visualize yourself relaxing more profound and deeper until you find yourself in a deep state of relaxation and ready to engage in a hypnotic visualization session.

Beginning with ten, visualize yourself taking a step down the stairs. Notice your surroundings, including the walls' color, what the bottom step looks like, and any decorations surrounding you. With nine, step down again, and see yourself getting closer to the bottom of the flight of stairs. Notice your relaxation doubling with every single step you take as you step down to the eighth step. Notice how your perspective may be changing around you as you descend lower and lower down the stairs, moving down to the seventh stair. Now, step down to the sixth stair. When you are ready, step again down to the fifth stair, feeling your relaxation doubling once again as you sink deeper and deeper into a state of relaxation and calmness. Now, step down to the fourth stair. As you look before you, you can see a chair coming into your view when you step down again to the third stair. As you step down to the second stair, you can see that the chair looks incredibly comfy, and you cannot wait to feel your relaxation triple when you sit in it as you step down to the first stair and then off the stairs.

When you get off the stairs at the bottom, see yourself walking up to that chair and sitting in it. Notice that this chair is the comfiest chair you have ever sat in, and upon sitting in it, you feel your entire state relaxing ten times deeper as you sink into the chair. Feel yourself becoming so calm that you can simply fade away in this space.

As you sit there, notice your awareness turning inward into your body. As your attention turns inward, draw your focus down into your fat cells. You sit there, hugging your body and keeping you warm and comfortable in your current state. Notice how each section feels confident that it is serving a purpose and sits proudly in its position. As you look at each of these fat cells, realize that they are not there to cause you harm or destruction, but because they genuinely believe they mean to be there. They think they are serving an essential job for you and your life.

As you draw your awareness even closer into these cells, I want you to pick one up in your hand. See this small round cell sitting in your hand, proudly serving a purpose in your life. As you hold it, thank the cell for all that it has done, and with complete gratitude, let it know that you no longer need it to help you anymore. Cup the section between your hands and feel it shrinking down until it vanishes between your palms.

Again, pick up another cell and hold it in your hands. With deep gratitude in your heart, thank it for serving its purpose and let it know that you no longer need its help. Wish it well as you cup it between your palms and shrink it down until it vanishes.

Keep doing this with your fat cells as you continue to pick them up, express gratitude for their service, and then shrink them down in your palms until they vanish entirely. One by one, let each fat cell know that it is no longer needed and that you are grateful for all that it has provided you with until this point in your life. Let your remaining cells know that you now require less fat in your body so that you can restore your health and start to feel better and better.

As you get to the end of the fat cells, notice that you look around and no fat cells remain. All you see are healthy cells that support essential functions in your body like cell regrowth, digestion, and circulation. Express deep gratitude for every cell in your body and its work, and allow yourself to release this perspective as you draw your awareness back into your body. See your awareness growing beyond the size of your small cells and back into the understanding of yourself as you come back into the room where you presently sit. Feel yourself awakening from your meditation now, as you open your eyes and feel different within your body.

From now on, when you go through your daily life, notice how even though some of your fat cells continue to remain, you can almost see them disappearing. Continue to express gratitude and all that it has done to attempt to support your survival and allow it to peacefully fade away as you allow yourself to come back into a state of poor health.

Meditation for Cutting Calories

This meditation is an excellent meditation to cut calories, allowing you to decrease the amount of food you are eating daily. It is a 10-15-minute meditation that will help you reduce cravings while also reducing your food intake daily. The purpose of this particular meditation is to reduce calorie intake without making you feel hungry, so the ultimate goal is to help you choose healthier meals, make you feel full, and reduce snacks between meals. You should engage in this meditation at the beginning of the day or any time you feel yourself experiencing difficulty with food cravings or moderation. That way, you can encourage yourself to stay on track with your weight loss goals. With that says, you should make sure that you are sitting up with a straight spine during this particular meditation so that you stay engaged and do not lose your energy or motivation following this specific meditation.

Start this meditation by sitting upright in a comfortable position with your spine long and tall and your awareness soft and gentle. When you are ready, I want you to begin to draw your attention to the center of your chest, directly behind your sternum. As you do, notice how it rises and falls with each breath you take. As you breathe in, feel your sternum pushing away from your spine, and as you breathe out, feel it falling back toward your spine. Continue to focus on this space for four breaths as you relax into this position and enjoy your meditation.

When you start to feel yourself relaxing, I want you to start visualizing yourself and putting together a meal. Start with breakfast. See yourself filling your plate with healthy options that fill you up without wasting calories. Notice how easy it is to fill your container with healthy things for you, which helps you feel your best. Allow yourself to begin feeling excited about the food options on that plate, noticing that you are genuinely craving them and looking forward to this meal. Visualize yourself taking a bite of the food and imagine how amazing it tastes. Notice how you feel yourself being completely satisfied with this food and that you do not have any reason to snack on anything in between because you are so content with the meal.

When it does come time to have a snack, or your next meal, see yourself having the desire to indulge in something healthy again. Notice how easy it is for you to pass up on junk foods or foods that do not support your health because you genuinely enjoy eating more beneficial things for you. See yourself readily opting for healthier food choices and enjoying each food option that you choose. Feel how great it is that being healthy, cutting calories, and losing weight can be delicious.

Now, when you are ready, bring your consciousness back into your current body. Feel yourself awakening into your body, coming back into your conscious state of awareness. Feel yourself effortlessly gravitating toward healthier meal options all day as you focus more on what will help you feel healthy, satisfied, and fulfilled from your meals.

CHAPTER 26:

Increase Your Wellbeing
With 150 Positive Affirmations

1. My beliefs shape my reality.

2. I realize that I'm the creator of my life.

3. I decide to make my life a masterpiece.

4. I know that if I believe it, I can see it.

5. I give and receive.

6. I'm grateful for the lessons my past has given me.

7. I'm a great giver; I'm also a great receiver.

8. I understand that my abundance of money can make the world a better place.

9. The universe responds to my mindset of abundance by giving me more prosperity.

10. I define my dream and feel gratitude for its realization.

11. I visualize living my dream every day.

12. I send out good vibrations about money.

13. I'm abundant in every way.

14. I'm grateful for all the money that I have. I'm grateful for all the prosperity that I receive.

15. I'm grateful for the present moment and focus on the beauty of life.

16. I pay myself first and make my money multiply.

17. I have a millionaire mind, and I now understand the principles behind wealth.

18. I love the freedom that money gives me.

19. I'm a multi-millionaire.

20. I choose to be me and free.

21. There is an infinite amount of opportunities for creating wealth in the world.

22. I see opportunities for creating wealth and act on them.

23. My motto is to act and adapt.

24. The answers always seem to come to me.

25. I have an attitude of gratitude.

26. I deserve to become wealthy.

27. I deserve to have the best in life.

28. I'm a wonderful person with patience.

29. I trust the universe to guide me to my true calling in life. Knowing this, I get a feeling of calmness.

30. I know that I'm becoming the best I can possibly be.

31. I feel connected to prosperity.

32. I love money and realize all the great things it can do.

33. I'm at one with a tremendous amount of money.

34. Money loves me, and therefore it will keep flowing to me.

35. I use my income wisely and always have a big surplus of money at the end of the month.

36. I truly love the feeling of being wealthy. I enjoy the freedom it gives me.

37. It is easy for me to understand how money works.

38. I choose to think in ways that support me in my happiness and success.

39. I'm an exceptional manager of money.

40. I realize that success in anything leaves clues.

41. I follow the formula of people who have created a fortune.

42. I create a lot of value for others.

43. I'm a valuable person.

44. My life is full of abundance.

45. I know about the 80 20 rule, which states that 80 % of the effects come from 20 % of the causes.

46. 20 % of my activities produce 80 % of the results.

47. I choose to focus on the most important things in my life.

48. I choose to become wealthy.

49. I make my money multiply by investing them wisely.

50. I pay myself first. 10 % of my income works for me.

51. Money works for me.

52. I increase my ability to earn by setting concrete goals and work to achieve them.

53. By implementing in my life the 80 20 rules, I increase my productivity and profitability.

54. I focus on the most important areas in my life and eliminate, delegate, or automate the rest.

55. Time is on my side now.

For Self-Love

56. I am totally worthy of love.

57. I am in love with myself for who and what I am.

58. I deserve unconditional love and happiness.

59. I am always surrounded by loving, caring, and nurturing people in life.

60. I am responsible for my happiness, and I love myself.

61. I am worthy of receiving a lot of love.

62. I've created a home filled with love, happiness, harmony, and joy.

63. The greater love I give, the more love I receive in return.

64. I am eternally grateful for every relationship and experience in my life.

65. I am a loving, giving, and forgiving person.

66. I treat the one I love with love, affection, and respect.

67. I am truly worthy of love, and I deserve to be loved and respected.

68. I am in love with a person who adores me.

69. I love and accept other people as they are, which creates lasting relationships/friendships for me.

70. I am loved, desired, and cherished.

71. My relationships are filled with desire, love, passion, fun, care, and understanding.

72. I cherish all my emotions and feelings.

73. I attract the perfect partner who satisfies my needs in an inspiring and positive manner.

74. I am highly sensitive to the needs of other people I am surrounded by.

75. I am surrounded by love, respect, and gratitude.

76. I am in a loving, respectful, and passionate relationship.

77. I am loving and being loved all the time.

78. I am grateful for all the love enveloping my life.

79. I give and get love effortlessly and easily.

80. The person I love is with me always, and the flow of love in our life only increases.

81. All the love I desire is within me.

82. I am loved and capable of giving love.

83. I am right now in a perfect relationship with a perfect partner.

84. I am surrounded by love all the time.

85. All my relationships are positive, caring, loving, inspiring, and long-term.

86. I am truly worthy of being loved and deserve to receive love in absolute abundance.

87. I love everyone around me, and others shower me with an abundance of love.

88. I always attract loving and caring people in life.

89. My partner and I are both in love and happy. Our relationship is truly glorious and joyous.

90. I attract loving, inspiring, caring, and positive people in my life.

91. I am thankful to the Universe for a loving and caring partner.

92. I have complete gratitude for attracting only healthy, loving, and positive relationships.

93. I am blessed to be with the love of my life. We treat each other with love, appreciation, and respect.

94. I happily attract and give love each day.

95. I am eternally grateful to my partner for how caring, positive, inspiring, and nurturing they are.

96. Every day, I am grateful for being loved and for receiving the care that I do.

97. I completely trust that the Universe will bring me supporting, loving, caring, inspiring, and positive relationships.

98. I open my heart to the knowledge that I deserve love.

99. Wherever I go, and whoever I am with, I will always find love.

100. I totally deserve the love I receive, and I am open to the love the Universe bestows upon me.

101. I am attracted to love, and romance, and love and romance are attracted to me.

102. I spread love and receive it several times over.

103. I trust the Universe will help me find my perfect soul mate.

104. I can feel and experience the love of those surrounding me immensely.

105. I love each and every aspect of my wonderful life.

106. Love fills my heart, body, and soul with warmth every day.

107. I become more loving, caring, and inspiring with each passing day.

108. Everything I do completely aligns with the vibration and frequency of love.

109. I give and receive love joyfully, amazingly, and freely.

110. My life is truly amazing because I find love everywhere I go. I enjoy being with people who bring out the best in me.

111. I love being with folks who bring out my best side.

112. I see myself as a creature of love, happiness, passion, and joy.

113. I am loved and accepted. I am loved and accepted. I am loved and accepted.

114. I matter because I contribute love to this world in a wonderful and meaningful manner.

115. My partner and I are a true reflection of each other.

116. I create a sanctuary within my house that is forever inviting and welcoming to my partner.

117. I stand firm, strong, and grounded in my love.

118. Love originates from my core existence and impacts all areas of my life.

119. I think positively and in a nurturing way about my partner.

120. I encourage my partner to aim for the stars.

121. My energy converts conflict into a sense of unity, alignment, and oneness.

122. I am content, happy, and joyful alone, and my partner just adds to the wonderful feeling that already exists.

123. I enjoy having fulfilling, rewarding, and nurturing relationships with my friends and family members.

124. I attract more and appreciate the joy of giving and getting unconditional love.

125. I seek the love of my life, and the love of my life seeks me.

126. I am grateful for the romance and love that I am attracting in my life.

127. I speak, think, and behave from a place of love within me.

128. I spend time with a person who unconditionally accepts me as I am.

129. I wholeheartedly welcome the romance and passion gushing into my life.

130. My relationship grows stronger, more passionate, and romantic each day.

131. Emotional intimacy is an integral part of my relationship each day.

132. My relationship grows stronger each day, and my love grows much deeper.

133. I am blessed to be in love with a person who is my true soul mate.

134. I am so happy and grateful now that my outlook on life is positive.

135. Being happy is easy for me.

136. I am grateful for every moment of every day because I know it will never come back.

137. My future is bright, and I am so thankful for it.

138. I think uplifting thoughts.

139. Life is easy for me.

140. I am thankful for my breath.

141. I always have what I need, and for that, I'm grateful.

142. I start every day in a state of happiness and joy.

143. I am a joyful giver and a happy receiver of good things in my life.

144. I am meant to be here in this world and fulfil a purpose.

145. The world will be a better and happier place because I was here.

146. I am an unstoppable force for good.

147. I trust myself; my inner wisdom knows the truth.

148. I forgive myself and others for all the mistakes I made.

149. I breathe in happiness with every breath I take.

150. This day brings me happiness.

CHAPTER 27:

The Most Effective Foods to Eat to Help You Lose Weight and Feel More Satisfied

Seek advice from a healthcare professional or registered dietitian prior to actually starting a new eating plan.

- **Low-calorie diets:** Reducing your daily calories by less than 1400 calories per day would be detrimental because your body adapts to a semi-hungry state and is looking for alternative energy sources. Your body eventually burns muscle tissue, in addition to fat burning. But since your heart is a muscle, it will be seriously damaged by times of starvation and tamper with its regular beats. Low-calorie foods do not satisfy the dietary requirements of the body, and the body can't function properly, lacking nutrition.

- **Appetite-suppressant medicines and other diet pills:** "Wonder" items that irreversibly promote weight loss don't really prevail. Goods that guarantee instant or unobtrusive loss of weight would not work long term. Satiety suppressants that often contain a psychoactive drug such as caffeine are associated with health risks such as morning sickness, nasal dryness, agitation, anxiety, lightheadedness, sleeplessness, and higher blood pressure.

- **Fad diets:** Most fad diets promote consuming a lot of one form of food instead of a range of foods, which may be very harmful. Such forms of diets are also designed to manipulate consumers into wasting more on unhealthy and even unproven goods. The best approach to consume requires balanced meals, so you can receive all the nutrition the body needs.

- **Liquid diets:** liquid dietary products or shakes that contain fewer than 1000 calories a day could be used under very strict professional monitoring. Such foods may be unhealthy and are not nutrient effective due to excessive amounts of sugar. There is also a very poor fibre content that induces blood sugar spikes and drops. Moreover, liquid diets do not reduce appetite, leading to the over-consumption of certain foods.

The Best Diet Approach for Healthy Weight Loss

Pick up every diet book, and it would falsely claim to contain all the keys to easily shed all the pounds you would like—and keep it all off. Many say that the trick is to consume less and workout more, some that fat-free is the only way to get there, and some recommend leaving out carbohydrates.

The irony is that there is no "one size fits all" approach for successful, safe weight reduction. What works with one individual does not work for another because our bodies adapt differently to specific diets, based on biology and other health considerations. It is possible that choosing the best weight loss strategy for you would take time and include persistence, determination, and also some exploration with multiple diets.

Although some people react well to calorie counting or similar restrictive techniques, others react favorably to getting more liberty in organizing their weight-loss strategies. Simply avoiding fried foods or cutting back on processed carbohydrates could even set them up to succeed. So, don't be too downhearted if a regimen that worked for someone else doesn't work for you.

Remember: although there's no obvious answer to lose weight, there are still plenty of measures that can be taken to establish a healthful attitude towards food, reduce binge eating emotional triggers and sustain a healthy weight.

Keeping the Weight Off

You might have noticed the commonly cited figures that 95 percent of people trying to lose weight on a diet can recover it within a matter of years—or even months. Although there are not any concrete data to confirm this argument, it's clear that many weight-loss programs struggle in the long term. Maybe it's probably because overly stringent diets are really challenging to manage over time. The (NWCR) National Weight Control Registry in the United States, since it was founded in 1994, has monitored over 10,000 people that have gained considerable quantities of weight and held it off over lengthy periods of time. The research showed that participants who have been effective in retaining their weight loss follow similar approaches.

- Stay fit and active. Prosperous dieters in the NWCR study exercise are typically going to walk for around 60 min.

- Keep a food log. Recording your daily intake helps to keep you responsible and driven.

- Consume breakfast every day. It's most often cereal and fruit in the research. Consuming breakfast increases the appetite, warding off cravings later that same day.

- Have more fiber than the standard American diet and less fat.

- Check your scale regularly. Trying to weigh yourself weekly may help you spot any slight weight gains, allowing you to take appropriate corrective actions even before a problem occurs.

- Watch less TV. Minimizing the hours spent sat in front of the television will be a vital aspect of having a healthier lifestyle and weight gain avoidance.

Hindrances in Weight Loss

Relying Too Much on Water

Drinking water is fantastic for the body. Although it is also claimed that consuming additional water then you'll need to ward off thirst is a magical weight losing trick—specifically consuming 6 to 8 glasses every day or more. Nevertheless, there is little confirmation that this will be effective. This turned out that drinking water, whether warm or room temperature, just expends a small number of calories. So focusing on this plan will not get you far from shedding pounds. On the other hand, people occasionally eat when they are really thirsty. And it is not a poor thing to quench the thirst before having a bite. It's always effective to approach for a drink of water than just a sugary drink, Pepsi or spice latte—any calorie drink can influence your quality of life, so there's no reason to think about it with water.

Sleeping Too Little—or Too Much

People put on some weight occasionally, for unexpected reasons. One in four Americans isn't having enough time. And it could be that the shortage of sleep contributes to the obesity problem. Dozens of scientific studies have explored a link between obesity and sleep in infancy, and several have identified a linkage. It is not clear if obesity makes it more difficult to have enough sleep or if sleep is what induces obesity. Many reports also aimed at people who are overweight. Such findings also indicate a correlation between increasing weight and getting more than 9 hours of sleep or below five hours. This could be due to hormone levels. Sleep cycles influence hormones linked to hunger and energy intake-burning-leptin and ghrelin. Besides that, individuals who sleep less generally feel fatigued and far less able to do workouts. If you have difficulty losing weight, you can focus on the quality of your sleep.

Relying on Restaurant Meals

Whether you have a full life or simply aren't a lover of home cooking, you place your body at the hands of the restaurants you buy from. Also, dishes marketed as "sweet" can contain more calories than you've been shopping for, so several restaurants, especially smaller ones, don't mention their nutritional statistics, so you can't see what you're really consuming. There's even evidence that people who eat restaurant lunches outweigh those who prepare lunch at home by an average of five pounds.

Too Many Tiny Meals

You might have got to hear that trying to eat lots of small meal options all day long helps keep you fuller for longer without any excess calories. Yet to confirm this, there is barely any statistical evidence. Not only they are tiny, but daily meals are also stressful for preparing, but they may potentially end up backfiring, forcing you to consume more, and then once you start feeding, it may be hard to quit. If that is how you want to fuel your body, go for it. But it doesn't matter if your restricted-calorie diet is ingested all day long or just three or four times a day. The most crucial part is having to eat a healthy diet with the proper calorie count.

Taking a Seat—All Day Long

Will that sound familiar to you? You are riding in the car to work and going to a workplace where you are working for much of the day. You're worn out when you get home and just want to—can you guess? Only sit down, maybe watch some television. All that sitting means your body doesn't move as much as it should for the best outcomes for your health. Studies have shown that those who spend more time sitting are more likely to weigh. But some studies say weighing more will lead people to sit more frequently. It's a complex process that affects the other, but here's something that's well known: while you're sitting, you're not driving, doing housework, or standing and running around a ton. All this energy that should be used by consuming a few more calories through exercise makes health suffer only with rest. And you can only benefit if you take out more space every day to exercise.

Overdoing Alcohol

Alcoholic beverages can expand your middle section more than you know. A beer or two a day is popular among many Americans. But it sure does add up. Anyone that consumes two shots of vodka a day per week contributes about 1,400 calories to their diet—that's most calories in a day! And add still more wine and beer. Two bottles of wine a week contribute about 1,600 calories to the weekly count, and about 2,100 beers a day. So if you're willing to get serious about weight loss, consider putting down the mug of beer for a while.

Rewarding Exercise with Food

Some people think that they can justify the extra help of pasta at dinner by working out. That may not, however, be the case. When we work out, we tend to overestimate the calories that we burn, and technology doesn't help. Researchers find in one analysis that the typical aerobic unit overestimates on typical calories burnt by 19 per cent. In that research, elliptical machines were the worst offenders, an average of 42 percent overestimating. That adds up to over a year's work out! Fitness bands have shown identical issues.

Turning to Snacks When You're Stressed Out

Have you ever learned of emotional eating? Eating can become an effort to fill an emotional vacancy within your life when you're stressed out. Sometimes this includes excessive snacking on high-calorie products, piling on pounds. One study had hair locks investigated for the cortisol stress hormone. For candidates who showed signs of long-term stress, they found a significant relationship between waist size and high body-mass index (BMI). None of this has a bright side to it. You can ease stress without having your wardrobe stretched out. Exercising can be the best way to both burn stress and lose weight. And relaxing techniques such as meditation, yoga, deep breathing, and massage can bring peace to your life—no calories needed.

CHAPTER 28:

How to Maintain Mindful Eating Habits in Your Life

Indeed, even with the best program and all the help on the planet, we as a whole have days when we could utilize some additional motivation. Here are a few things you can do to build your inspiration and assurance of your weight reduction achievement.

Set Achievable Goals

Something I can't pressure enough is the significance of making changes that you will have the option to stay with for an amazing remainder.

Start by defining little reachable objectives that aren't attached to a number on a scale. For model, rather than making it your objective to lose 10 kilos, why not intend to drink eight glasses of water each day. Or then again, plan to take the stairs every morning on your approach to work. Another very accommodating objective is to tune in to your entrancing chronicles, in any event, four times each week.

Whatever your objectives, ensure they are quite certain, unmistakable, and simple to achieve.

To move more and have activity is critical to wellbeing, and when you are attempting to shed pounds, it makes a difference like never before. Be that as it may, it is anything but difficult to get exhausted with the regular old exercise schedule for quite a while. Try not to stall out stuck!

Have a go at something new. Take a walk, take a yoga class, or investigate your neighborhood with a morning climb.

Exercise doesn't need to be done in a rec center, on a bit of gear, or with a teacher. You simply need to get going!

Prepare for the New You

Prepare for the new form of yourself that you are making. You must wipe out any unfortunate nourishment from the cabinets. Dispose of old garments from the wardrobe. Modify your condition to suit the new life you are building.

Try not to Give in to Guilt

Nobody is immaculate, and we, as a whole, need a little chocolate sometimes. The main thing amiss with the infrequent guilty pleasure is the blame you feel a short time later. There is no point making yourself feel so awful about that one binge to spend that it thumps you totally off track, and you wind up eating ten chocolates just to feel good. Normally thin individuals don't feel regretful when they have a periodic treat. They relish the experience and afterward get directly back to eating well nourishments. Blame isn't valuable—let it go!

Kevin's Story Seeing the Hidden Price Tag for Unhealthy Food

Kevin was a foodie. He wanted to eat. He additionally adored biking and drinking wine. Be that as it may, those three things didn't appear to go together very well since he regularly drank excessively a lot of wine and didn't want to ride, and in addition to he had an additional 15 pounds he had been attempting to shed throughout the previous five years. The additional weight made him riding with his friends harder, and he hadn't had a ton of fun as of late for that very reason.

He came in for trance since he needed to curtail his drinking and gorging, get in shape, and become a superior cyclist.

Kevin's issue was not quite the same as Patty's: he could go for quite a long time without nourishment, regularly working through lunch, and having very late meals. Yet, he likewise accepted an existence without great wine, cheddar, and the pastry wasn't one worth living. He really had an image in his mind of himself getting a charge out of wine, cheddar, and pastry with friends after a decent ride, and his bicycle was out of sight of this image. This was a picture he made that speaks to his optimal life, and it fulfilled him to consider it. It likewise was a piece of what was making him over-enjoy in light of the fact that Kevin wasn't seeing the full picture—the genuine expense of what an overindulgence of high-caloric nourishments and liquor was doing to his body. For Kevin, it wasn't as a lot of a constraining conviction as it was not seeing reality with regards to the decisions he was making.

Mesmerizing can assist us with distinguishing and be freed of restricting convictions on account of Patty and Jessie; however, it can likewise assist us with seeing things for how they really are. What's more, to explain, when I state "see things," what I mean is that individuals are envisioning something in their brain—regardless of whether they're seeing it or simply thinking about it. Not every person really makes pictures in their mind.

I will use "see" until further notice. For certain individuals, considering things as they really imply as opposed to considering what a threat is, as something that satisfies them, they consider it as something that satisfies them for 10 minutes, at which point, they feel responsible and regret it for the rest of the day. It implies seeing a glass of wine not as a pressure reliever, yet as a depressant that is really noxious to their body. A few eaters will really change the image in their minds. They imagine their favorite bag of candy with a puckered face or an image of genuine, heavier spending. Since that is an increasingly exact picture of what the treats will do, imagine a scenario where makers were required to put outwardly of items what truly happened in the wake of expending them. Well, will you buy a package of chips with a picture of an overweight, dejected person watching TV on the front? Shouldn't something be said about candy with a picture of an overweight, dejected individual on the outside? Also, shouldn't something be said about that pack of nourishment from the drive-through or take out—an image of you feeling worn out and drowsy?

The next time you buy an item, imagine that the package has a picture of you 15 minutes after it is used. See how that changes things for you. That's true in advertising.

The mind helped Kevin to concentrate and pay attention to understand what he was really doing; in case he enjoyed the taste of food and wine so much, was a second or third glass really vital? Is it correct to say that it was even that big glass constantly? True wine authorities spit out their wine after tasting it. Shouldn't something be said about eating the whole piece of your favorite cheesecake, that that tenth bite was on par with the first?

Kevin understood the genuine expense of his extreme drinking—it was constraining his profitability at work, and it was shielding him from being a superior cyclist. He understood in the event that he genuinely cherished the flavor of wine, one glass would be sufficient. More than that, and he may have an alternate issue.

Portioning Your Food

1. Toss Out Your Scales

Do you think thin individuals bounce on the scales each morning? No, they don't. Fixating on the scales makes you a captive to them. At the point when you lose a pound or two, you may feel extraordinary, yet in the event that you increase a little, at that point, it can set you into a winding of implosion. The sentiments of disappointment that you pursue can send you running for the closest bar of chocolate or other solace food.

Also, restroom scales are not a precise method to screen your weight. Imagine a scenario where you are practicing more and picking up muscle. Or then again, perhaps you need a decent solid discharge — well, there goes a couple of additional pounds? Women, is it that time, and your body is puffed up with liquid weight? Such a large number of components can impact that number on the scales.

So, it's a great opportunity to quit making a decision about your prosperity by what you gauge and start taking a gander at all the positive changes you are making in your life. Give it a chance to feel, and the good decisions you make, be your new weight reduction indicator. Or, on the other hand, essentially watch as your garments get looser and your body gets littler.

2. Tune in to Your Body

Pause for a minute or two to inquire as to whether you feel extremely eager. There are some common signs when we think we feel hungry, however just not many when we are really eager.

Frequently we feed our sentiments as a result of a bogus enthusiastic craving. Or on the other hand, perhaps we botch feeling anxious for feeling hungry.

Genuine hunger is that slight chewing or void sensation in your stomach. Set aside an effort to tune in to your body, to truly tune in to your body's needs. Eat possibly to fulfill genuine craving and stop when your body has had enough. Pick food sources that make you feel fulfilled, supported, and light, and keep away from all nourishments that make you feel substantial, enlarged, and awkward. It's as straightforward as that!

3. Bite Your Food

Processing starts in your mouth, and great assimilation is basic to changing the food you eat into the vitality your body needs. When you bite into your food, it invigorates the discharge of digestion-related acids into your stomach and related tract. In the event that you eat too rapidly, these proteins don't have the opportunity they have to process your nourishment viably. At the point when you eat rapidly, you likewise swallow more air and ingest bigger parts of food, which puts a strain on your stomach related framework and can cause swelling and gas.

Additionally, the appetite hormone Leptin will keep on expanding as you eat until your hunger has been fulfilled. Biting your food altogether and gradually eating gives your body time to perceive that it is full and permits leptin to communicate something specific from your stomach to your cerebrum to quit eating since you have had enough.

4. Eat Smaller Meals More Often

Eat no less than each 4-5 hours to give your body the fuel it needs to work effectively. This will help keep up your glucose levels and keep your digestion firing up. Plan ahead with the goal that you have good nourishment close by persistence. Keep in mind that you need to eat when you begin to feel hungry, not after you become covetous. At the point when you experience over the top appetite, it is an indication of low glucose levels, which will make longings for sugar and other CRAP food.

5. Make the Most of Your Food

Go down, slow down, relax, and make the most of your power. Making a relaxed and charming atmosphere when you eat encourages you to bite more completely, eat more gradually, and make it easier to tune in to your body. In the same way, try to abstain from anything that occupies your consideration away from eating, for example, sitting in front of the television. Along these lines, you are bound to stay mindful of the amount you are eating. The more cognizant you are of the point at which you are eating, the more you will tune in to the sign saying you have had enough.

CHAPTER 29:

Blasting Calories

We have all heard the word "calorie" and its relation to our body weight—calories contained in the foods we consume and often misunderstood about how they affect us. We seek to explain what they are, how to count them, and the best methods of blasting them to avoid weight gain.

What Are Calories and How They Affect Your Weight

A calorie is a fundamental estimating unit. For example, we use meters when communicating separation; "Usain Bolt went 100 meters in merely 9.5 seconds." There are two units in this expression. One is a meter (a range unit), and the other is "second" (a period unit). Necessarily, calories are additional units of substantial amount estimation.

Many assume that a calorie is the weight measure (since it is frequently connected with an individual's weight). That is not precise, however. A calorie is a vitality unit (estimation). One calorie is proportional to the vitality expected to build the temperature by 1 degree Celsius to 1 liter of water.

Two particular sorts of calories come in: small calories and massive calories. Huge calories are the word connected to sustenance items.

You've likely observed much stuff on parcels (chocolates, potato chips, and so forth.) with "calorie scores." Imagine the calorie score as an incentive for a thing being "100 cal." this infers when you eat it, you will pick up about as much vitality (even though the calorie worth expressed and the amount you advantage from it is never the equivalent).

All we eat has a particular calorie tally; it is the proportion of the vitality we eat in the substance bonds.

These are mostly things we eat: starches, proteins, and fats. How about we take a gander at what number of calories 1 gram comprises of these meals: 1. Sugars, four calories 2. Protein, three calories. Fat, nine calories.

My Are Calories Awful

That is fundamentally equivalent to mentioning, "Is vitality awful for me?" Every single activity the body completes needs vitality. Everything takes energy to stand, walk, run, sit, and even eat. In case you're doing any of these tasks, it suggests you're utilizing vitality, which mostly infers you're' consuming' calories, explicitly the calories that entered your body when you were eating some food.

To sum things up, for you, NO... calories are not terrible.

Equalization is the way to find harmony between the number of calories you devour and what number of calories you consume. On the off chance that you eat fewer calories and spend more, you will become dainty. In contrast, on the opposite side, on the off chance that you gobble up heaps of calories, however, you are a habitually lazy person. You will, in the long run, become stout at last.

Each movement we do throughout a day will bring about sure calories spent. Here is a little rundown of the absolute most much of the time performed exercises, just as the number of calories consumed while doing them.

Step By Step Instructions to Count Calories

You have to expend fewer calories than you consume to get thinner.

This clamor is simple in principle. Be that as it may, it very well may be hard to deal with your nourishment admission in the contemporary sustenance setting. Calorie checking is one approach to address this issue and is much of the time used to get more fit. Hearing that calories don't make a difference is very common, and tallying calories is an exercise in futility. Nonetheless, calories tally with regards to weight; this is a reality in which, in science, analyses called overloading studies have demonstrated numerous occasions.

These investigations request that people deliberately indulge and, after that, survey the impact on their weight and wellbeing. All overloading investigations have found that people are putting on weight when they devour a more significant number of calories than they consume.

This simple reality infers that calorie checking and limiting your utilization can be proficient in averting weight put on or weight reduction as long as you can stick to it. One investigation found that health improvement plans, including calorie, brought about an average weight reduction of around 7 lbs. (3.3 kg) more than those that didn't.

Primary concern: You put on weight by eating a more significant number of calories than you consume. Calorie tallying can help you expend fewer calories and get more fit.

How many calories do you have to eat? What number of calories do you need depends on factors such as sex, age, weight, and measure of activity? In case you're endeavoring to get in shape, by eating not correctly your body consumes off, you'll have to construct a calorie deficiency. Utilize this adding machine to decide what number of calories you ought to expend every day (opening in crisp tab). This number cruncher depends on the condition of Mifflin-St Jeor, an exact method to evaluate calorie prerequisites.

How to Reduce your Caloric Intake for Weight Loss

Bit sizes have risen, and a solitary dinner may give twofold or triple what the regular individual needs in a sitting at certain cafés. "Segment mutilation" is the term used to depict huge parts of sustenance as the standard. It might bring about weight put on and weight reduction. In general, people don't evaluate the amount they spend. Tallying calories can help you battle indulging by giving you more grounded information about the amount you expend. In any case, you have to record portions of sustenance appropriately for it to work. Here are some well-known strategies for estimating segment sizes:

- **Scales:** Weighing your sustenance is the most exact approach to decide the amount you eat. This might be tedious, in any case, and isn't always down to earth.

- **Estimating cups:** Standard estimations of amount are, to some degree, quicker and less complex to use than a scale, yet can some of the time be tedious and unbalanced.

- **Investigations:** It's quick and easy to utilize correlations with popular items, especially in case you're away from home. It's considerably less exact, however.

Contrasted with family unit items, here are some mainstream serving sizes that can gauge your serving sizes: 1 serving of rice or pasta (1/2 a cup): the size of a PC mouse or adjusted bunch.

- 1 Meat serving (3 oz): a card deck

- 1 Fish serving (3 oz): visit book

- 1 Cheese serving (1.5 oz): a lipstick or thumb size

- 1 Fresh organic product serving (1/2 cup): a tennis ball

- 1 Green verdant vegetable serving (1 cup): baseball

- 1 Vegetable serving (1/2 cup): a mouse PC

- 1 Olive oil teaspoon: 1 fingertip

- 2 Peanut margarine tablespoons: a ping pong ball

Calorie tallying, notwithstanding when gauging and estimating partitions, isn't an exact science.

In any case, your estimations shouldn't be thoroughly spot-on. Simply guarantee that your utilization is recorded as effectively as would be prudent. You should be mindful of marking high-fat as well as sugar things, for example, pizza, dessert, and oils. Under-recording these meals can make an enormous qualification between your genuine and recorded utilization. You can endeavor to utilize scales toward the beginning to give you an excellent idea of what a segment resembles to upgrade your evaluations. This should help you to be increasingly exact, even after you quit utilizing them.

More Tips to Assist in Caloric Control

Here are five more calorie tallying tips:

- **Get prepared:** get a calorie counting application or web device before you start, choose how to evaluate or gauge parcels, and make a feast plan.

- **Read nourishment marks:** Food names contain numerous accommodating calorie tallying information. Check the recommended segment size on the bundle.

- **Remove the allurement:** Dispose of your home's low-quality nourishment. This will help you select more advantageous bites and make hitting your objectives easier.

- **Aim for moderate, steady loss of weight; don't cut too little calories:** Even though you will get in shape all the more rapidly, you may feel terrible and be less inclined to adhere to your arrangement.

- **Fuel your activity:** Diet and exercise are the best health improvement plans. Ensure you eat enough to rehearse your vitality.

Effective Methods for Blasting Calories

To impact calories requires participating in exercises that urge the body to utilize vitality. Aside from checking the calories and guaranteeing you eat the required amount, consuming them is similarly essential for weight reduction. Here, we examine a couple of techniques that can enable you to impact our calories all the more viably:

- **Indoor cycling:** McCall states that around 952 calories for each hour should be 200 watts or higher. On the off chance that the stationary bicycle doesn't demonstrate watts: "this infers you're doing it when your indoor cycling instructor educates you to switch the opposition up!" he proposes.

- **Skiing:** Around 850 calories for every hour depends on your skiing knowledge. Slow, light exertion won't consume nearly the same number of calories as a lively, fiery effort wasted. To challenge yourself and to consume vitality? Attempt to ski tough.

- **Rowing:** Approximately consumes 816 calories for every hour. The benchmark here is 200 watts; McCall claims it ought to be at a "fiery endeavor." many paddling machines list the showcase watts. Reward: rowing is additionally a stunning back exercise.

- **Jumping rope:** About 802 calories for each hour this ought to be at a moderate pace—around 100 skips for each moment—says McCall. Attempt to begin with this bounce rope interim exercise.

- **Kickboxing:** Approximately blasts 700 calories for every hour. Also, in this class are different sorts of hand to hand fighting, for example, Muay Thai with regards to standard boxing, when you are genuine in the ring (a.k.a. Battling another individual), the most significant calorie consumption develops. Be that as it may, many boxing courses add cardio activities, for example, hikers and burpees, so your pulse will, in the long run, increase more than you would anticipate. What's more, hello, before you can get into the ring, you need to start someplace, isn't that so?

- **Swimming:** Freestyle works approximately 680 calories per hour, however as McCall says, you should go for a vivacious 75 yards for each moment. For an easygoing swimmer, this is somewhat forceful. (butterfly stroke is significantly progressively productive if you extravagant it.)

- **Outdoor bicycling:** Approximately 680 calories for each hour biking at a fast, lively pace will raise your pulse, regardless of whether you are outside or inside. Add to some rocky landscape and mountains, and it gets significantly more calorie consuming.

The volume of calories devoured is straightforwardly proportionate to the measure of sustenance, just like the kind of nourishment an individual expends. The best way to lessen calories is by being cautious about what you devour and captivating in dynamic physical exercises to consume an overabundance of calories in your body.

CHAPTER 30:

Mental exercise

When we think of weight management, our minds often go-to diet and exercise. What's more important than hitting the gym is exercising our brain. If we make sure that the most important organ in our body is taken care of, we can be certain that other healthy habits will soon follow. You can diet, exercise, and do everything else you need to lose weight, but if you continually distract, deflect, or avoid your problems, you might not find the happiness you seek. The happier you feel, and the more you are aware of your mental health the better it will be in the end, which will also lead to overall better quality of life.

Keep a Journal

Keeping a journal is a healthy habit for many people, no matter what their goals are, but it's important for someone that wants to lose weight as well. By writing down your different portion measurements and exercise habits, you can better ensure that you'll have a basis for evaluation.

When this is done, you can predict future problems that might keep you from your goals by looking back on the days of recorded mistakes or slipups. You can see what kinds of schedules and structures aren't working so you can create better habits in the end. The more extensive your journaling, the better you'll be able to create your own research study of your weight-loss journey, meaning you can share your progress or use it as a structure for future diets.

Avoid the Scale

The biggest issue with weight-loss strugglers comes when they see the number on the scale. Someone that wants to lose ten pounds might get discouraged if they find they only lost nine. Sometimes, people might even have to gain weight before they end up losing a pound. By avoiding the scale altogether, certain failures and disappointments can be avoided as well.

Find a different way to track your progress. You can have monthly weigh-ins, but it shouldn't be something that should be checked once a day. Our weight fluctuates so much throughout our journey that it isn't worth stressing over on a daily basis. Any checking that happens more than once a day is also likely a bad habit; you're using it to distract yourself from a bigger issue.

The Calorie Myth

When many people diet, they focus too much on calories. They'll see that a certain snack pack only has a hundred calories, which means that it's good for you, right? Wrong. When we focus too much on how many calories are in something, we're failing to look at all the other factors that make up that product. Something with zero calories might include harmful chemicals or hidden substances that are bad for us. Something with a ton of calories might be avoided even though it has a large number of vitamins and necessary fiber.

Calories should still be considered, as the more calories you take in, the more you have to burn through exercise. They still shouldn't be a basis for what foods you decide to eat. If you focus too much on calories, you'll end up losing sight of other important issues. Remember that weight loss isn't about numbers. What's on the scale or on the nutrition package is important in making certain measurements, but they shouldn't be the definitive goals that you're creating on your weight-loss journey.

Talk About It

Keeping things indoors is never a good thing. In fact, it may seem horrible. Those who are overweight may feel embarrassed about their weight. They may end up apologizing for eating certain foods, verbalizing these reasons to those around them as a means of validation. "Oh, I'm going to start my diet tomorrow," someone can be heard saying as they pull out a few more cupcakes from the dessert table. This type of discussion can be contradictory. Instead, try to talk about the problems and difficulties you face, rather than how you will solve them later. You may find that you get good advice from someone who is facing a similar struggle.

It is also important to know how to listen. Sometimes people do not seek answers or advice when they complain about their problems. It's nice to have someone to vent to once in a while. By creating a discussion, you can more easily address the matters that are causing you problems on your journey to weight loss.

Avoid telling people about your goal before you get on track, however. Talking about your feelings, emotions, and struggles is always a good thing. Sometimes it just takes saying a thing out loud for it to feel real. However, many people set themselves up for failure by sharing their goals too early. Those that post on social media about how they're going to lose weight are actually less likely to follow through with their goals. Be quiet at the beginning of your journey, confiding in just those you know you can rely on and trust.

Affirmations

Practicing affirmations is an important mindset strategy in weight loss. An affirmation is a type of positive reinforcement that helps in combating negative thoughts. Instead of telling yourself, you're "no good" because you didn't follow through with a small goal, you should give yourself an affirmation such as "I am capable of continuing" to remind yourself of how powerful you really are. Below is a list of positive affirmations you should use in order to combat negative thoughts and improve overall encouragement:

1. I can do this. I am capable of losing weight, and I have the ability to reach my goals.

2. I am exercising every day and eating healthy as often as possible. I am actually doing what I should be doing in order to achieve my goals.

3. If I can start my journey, I can finish it.

4. I do not need processed foods to feel happy. I can feel the same joy from cooking a healthy meal.

5. I have exercised before and can do it again. It is hard to start, but I know that once I do, I have what it takes to finish my exercise routine.

6. I am healing myself. I have been through challenging times and deserve to feel happy.

7. I am loved and am full of love.

8. I am losing weight to be healthy.

9. I am beautiful no matter what size. Skipping one day at the gym does not mean that I am not beautiful.

10. I am eating healthy food full of nourishment. I can feel the positive change in my body, and I know that I only have more to look forward to.

Conclusion

If you have been disciplined enough to follow the meditation exercises we have covered in this book, you must have started seeing some real benefits. If you follow the instructions given in this meditation book, you can master everything and even start doing the exercises without having to look at the guidelines.

Whenever you find that you are stuck somewhere, and you do not know how to go with a particular meditation, you can always refer to this book and see what you need to do to move with the exercises smoothly. This book has a wealth of knowledge that you can use to achieve tremendous benefits when it comes to maintaining a healthy weight and the lifestyle you need to keep for a long time. Remember that it is not only about reducing your weight and achieving your weight goals. We first focused on weight reduction, and then we moved to other areas of life. After you have reached your desired goals with your weight, it is essential that you also look to other areas of your life and work on them.

The importance of focusing on other areas of your life is that you will maintain your weight goals for a long time. As we mentioned, there are many people who work hard only to reduce their weight, and once they are through with either the dieting program they had chosen or the meditation exercises they were doing, they quickly go back to their starting point, which means they gain the weight that they had lost. This is why I have covered these tips in this book because you should not go back to where you started. The best way to achieve this goal is to ensure that all areas of your life are functioning well. When these aspects are right, you are now able to have the strength that you need to maintain the current weight that you have achieved. The concept is that you need to remain in this state for the rest of your life since this makes you enjoy your presence to the fullest.

It is fair to say that this information is useful to you and many others who have considered using it in their program to control their weight. As you have discovered, meditation is a crucial tool that you can use in your daily life. Apart from that, it has helped you achieve the weight that you desire it can also help you in other areas of your life. This means that you can keep on practicing these meditation tips as long as you find them helpful and contributing positively to the growth and development of all angles of your life. For many years, those who have discovered the many benefits that come with meditation have been doing it for various reasons. Some do meditation for spiritual purposes, while others do it when faced with a lot of stress. Although many people have found help with meditation and many have solved their weight problem, this does not mean that everyone can gain the same results others have obtained. It largely depends on the effort that you put as an individual. Working hard will help you achieve this, which is why you find that maintaining focus has been emphasized a lot in this book.

What can you do if you find that you have done everything required for your meditation exercises, but still, you do not see any results? Honestly, some people say that meditation is not their thing, and they have tried it severally, yet it has not worked. If this is the experience you have had with the meditation exercises that we have covered in this book, you do not have to curse yourself. This may not be your problem since different people can get varying results with the mediation program they plan to use. Other ways are also useful, and you can use them to attain the healthy weight you want. It should not be the end of the road if it does not work for you. If you have found this useful and you are happy with the results that you gained, congratulations!

GASTRIC BAND HYPNOSIS EXTREME WEIGHT LOSS

Discover the Powerful Hypnotic Effect of Positive Affirmations.
Control Sugar Cravings and Weight Gain with
the Power of Meditation and Mindset Change

Introduction

The Gastric Band is a hypnosis process used to change the lives of seriously overweight and obese people who've been unsuccessful at reducing weight using other techniques. It replaces the actual Gastric Bypass Surgery with a hypnosis-based different focused on achieving the very same result of reducing the quantity of food the stomach can take in one meal. While this sort of surgery of the mind is not new, its weight loss application is unique.

Researchers worldwide agree that one of the keys to wellness, health, and individual growth depends on understanding the mind/body connection.

Gastric band hypnosis is more secure and less pricey than having the equivalent surgery executed.

The hypnotic gastric band system changes the size of your stomach, but it also helps you get comfortable and enjoy healthier foods. Hypnogastric banding is a healthier, longer-term, non-evasive option. Changing your body physically cannot give you long-term results, but you can enjoy healthier alternatives by tackling the main problem of over-eating.

Your body is a genuinely astonishing machine. It produces all the energy you use. It keeps your heart thumping and your lungs breathing two 4 hours every day. It does a lot from using only the food you eat, the air you inhale, and the energy it has put away in your body. Simultaneously it fixes and keeps up itself while never halting work.

When we fit your hypnotic gastric band, that fueling, fixing, and maintenance system keeps on working similarly as nature intends, however, there will be a couple of significant differences:

1. You will have less space for food in your stomach.

2. You will feel full sooner.

3. That "full" feeling will be urgent and easy to notice.

4. You are probably going to encounter changes in your food choices.

5. With the hypnotic band, there is no physical medical procedure, and therefore no physical dangers.

6. The hypnotic band is a less expensive

As you are eating less, your body might be pickier or search out new foods to guarantee it gets all the sustenance it requires. You don't need to stress over this with your conscious mind by any means. You keep on eating exactly what you need, but you'll see that what you need to eat changes. In the early stages, those progressions might be very subtle, so it might take you a little effort to understand that you currently find various foods more appealing.

The Magic of Your Digestive System

It will be useful to have a diagram of your digestive system with the goal that you see how your hypnotic gastric band functions. A few people are interested and keen on how the body functions; others are most certainly not. Notwithstanding, whatever you deliberately think, it is significant that you read this segment with the goal that your conscious mind has all the information it needs to process my hypnotic instructions. So regardless of whether you discover this segment somewhat complex, simply continue reading because your conscious mind will comprehend and use all it needs from this clarification.

Your digestive system begins functioning when you smell your food. Your salivary glands begin to secrete saliva when the food enters your mouth; saliva begins to blend in with it to make it simpler to swallow and to start to breakdown the diet. Next, the physical movement of chewing your food sends signals to your stomach to release hydrochloric acid. When you swallow, the food goes down your throat, or in medical terms, your esophagus. At the base of your throat is a solid valve called a sphincter, which unwinds to give the food access to your stomach. The sphincter shields your throat from the acid in your stomach. Sometimes, heartburn or overeating makes gastrointestinal reflux through that sphincter into your throat.

That builds up what we call indigestion. In your stomach, your food is blended in with acid and enzymes that break down the food into smaller particles. Proteins and fats take more time to process than sugars, so various foods take time to break down in the stomach. Vegetables do not take up to six0 minutes, and red meat can take a few hours to process. You don't need to worry about this, and your body does everything naturally.

From the stomach, your food, now broken down into micro pieces, is released bit by bit into your small intestine. Then, when the food goes into your intestines, your body extracts the nutrients for sustenance. Various enzymes further break it down into particles that are sufficiently small to pass through the walls of your intestines into the bloodstream. Carbohydrates are separated into glucose, which is taken to the liver. Glucose is used to control the muscles in your body. Proteins are separated into amino acids and sent into the bloodstream circulating all through the body and used to build and repair cells and tissues.

As the food goes through your small intestine, each of the nutrients is separated into various micro-molecules. In the colon, the water and salts that helped the process are absorbed once again into your body, and the rest is excreted. Every one of these processes is controlled by a lot of hormones, or signaling chemicals, in your body. In your digestive tract, one of the most important is called glucagon-like peptide-1 (known as glp-1). It is released as food enters your intestines. Glp-1 does loads of various jobs.

Since glp-1 does both these jobs at the same time, the feeling of fullness is connected to the process that gets energy into your muscles. This guarantees you don't feel full until your body is getting all the energy it needs. Levels of another hormone, called peptide yy (known as pyy), also increase when you have eaten. Pyy diminishes hunger and builds the capacity for nutrient absorption, so again it aids to signal you to stop eating to ensure you get what you need. Levels of a third hormone, called ghrelin, decline after a meal. Ghrelin is one of the hormones that cause us to feel hunger.

CHAPTER 1:

What it is Important to Know About Hypnosis

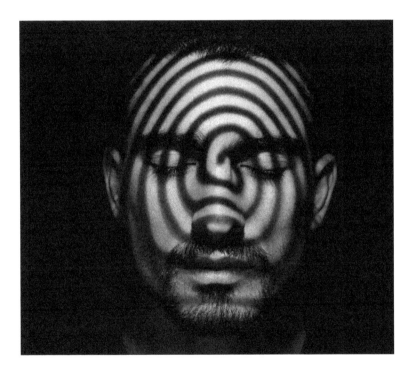

While brainwashing is a notable type of mind control that numerous individuals have about, hypnosis is additionally a significant sort that ought to be thought of. Generally, the individuals who know about hypnosis think about it from watching stage shows of members doing silly acts. While this is a sort of hypnosis, there is much more to it. This part is going to focus more on hypnosis as a type of mind control.

What Is Hypnosis?

To begin with, what is the meaning of hypnosis? As indicated by specialists, hypnosis is viewed as a condition of cognizance that includes the engaged consideration alongside the diminished fringe mindfulness that is described by the member's expanded ability to react to recommendations that are given. This implies the member will enter an alternate perspective and will be substantially more defenseless to following the recommendations that are given by the trance inducer.

It is broadly perceived that two hypothesis bunches help to depict what's going on during the hypnosis time frame. The first is the changing state hypothesis. The individuals who follow this hypothesis see that hypnosis resembles a daze or a perspective that is adjusted where the member will see that their mindfulness is, to some degree, not quite the same as what they would see in their common cognizant state. The other hypothesis is non-state speculations. The individuals who follow this hypothesis don't believe that the individuals who experience hypnosis are going into various conditions of awareness. Or maybe, the member is working with the subliminal specialist to enter a sort of inventive job authorization.

While in hypnosis, the member is thought to have more fixation and center that couples together with another capacity to focus on a particular memory or thought strongly. During this procedure, the member is likewise ready to shut out different sources that may be diverting to them. The mesmerizing subjects are thought to demonstrate an increased capacity to react to recommendations that are given to them, particularly when these proposals originate from the subliminal specialist. The procedure that is utilized to put the member into hypnosis is knitted hypnotic enlistment and will include a progression of proposals and guidelines that are utilized as a kind of warm-up.

There is a wide range of musings that are raised by specialists with regards to what the meaning of hypnosis is. The wide assortment of these definitions originates from the way that there are simply such huge numbers of various conditions that accompany hypnosis, and nobody individual has a similar encounter when they are experiencing it.

Some various perspectives and articulations have been made about hypnosis. A few people accept that hypnosis is genuine and are suspicious that the legislature and others around them will attempt to control their minds. Others don't have faith in hypnosis at all and feel that it is only skillful deception. No doubt, the possibility of hypnosis as mind control falls someplace in the center.

There are three phases of hypnosis that are perceived by the mental network. These three phases incorporate acceptance, recommendation, and defenselessness. Every one of them is critical to the hypnosis procedure and will be talked about further underneath.

Induction

The principal phase of hypnosis is induction. Before the member experiences the full hypnosis, they will be acquainted with the hypnotic enlistment method. For a long time, this was believed to be the strategy used to place the subject into their hypnotic stupor. However, that definition has changed some in current occasions. A portion of the non-state scholars has seen this stage somewhat in an unexpected way. Rather, they consider this to be the strategy to elevate the members' desires for what will occur, characterizing the job that they will play, standing out enough to be noticed to center the correct way, and any of the different advances that are required to lead the member into the correct heading for hypnosis.

There are a few induction procedures that can be utilized during hypnosis. The most notable and compelling strategies are Braid's "eye obsession" method or "Braidism." There are many varieties of this methodology, including the Stanford Hypnotic Susceptibility Scale

(SHSS). This scale is the most utilized instrument to examine in the field of hypnosis.

To utilize the Braid enlistment procedures, you should follow several means. The first is to take any object that you can find that is brilliant, for example, a watch case, and hold it between the centers, fore, and thumb fingers on the left hand. You will need to hold this item around 8-15 crawls from the eyes of the member. Hold the item someplace over the brow, so it creates a ton of strain on the eyelids and eyes during the procedure with the goal that the member can keep up a fixed gaze on the article consistently. The trance inducer should then disclose to the member that they should focus their eyes consistently on the article. The patient will likewise need to concentrate their mind on that specific item. They ought not to be permitted to consider different things or let their minds and eyes meander or, in all likelihood, the procedure won't be effective.

A little while later, the member's eyes will start to enlarge. With somewhat more time, the member will start to accept a wavy movement. If the member automatically shuts their eyelids when the center and forefingers of the correct hand are conveyed from the eyes to the item, at that point, they are in the stupor. If not, at that point, the member should start once more; make a point to tell the member that they are to permit their eyes to close once the fingers are conveyed in a comparable movement back towards the eyes once more. This will get the patient to go into the adjusted perspective that is knaps hypnosis.

While Braid remained by his method, he acknowledged that utilizing the acceptance procedure of hypnosis isn't constantly fundamental for each case. Analysts in current occasions have typically discovered that the acceptance strategy isn't as essential with the impacts of hypnotic recommendation as recently suspected. After some time, different other options and varieties of the first hypnotic acceptance procedure have been created, even though the Braid strategy is as yet thought about the best.

Recommendation

Present-day sleep induction utilizes a variety of proposal shapes to be fruitful, for example, representations, implications, roundabout or non-verbal recommendations, direct verbal proposals, and different metaphors and recommendations that are non-verbal. A portion of the non-verbal proposals that might be utilized during the recommendation stage would incorporate physical manipulation, voice tonality, and mental symbolism.

One of the qualifications that are made in the kinds of recommendation that can be offered to the member incorporates those proposals that are conveyed with consent and those that progressively tyrant in the way.

Something that must be considered concerning hypnosis is the contrast between the oblivious and the cognizant mind. There are a few trance specialists who see the phase of the proposal as a method of conveying that is generally guided to the cognizant mind of the subject. Others in the field will see it the other way; they see the correspondence happening between the operator and the subconscious or oblivious mind.

They accepted that the recommendations were being tended to directly to the conscious piece of the subject's mind, as opposed to the oblivious part. Braid goes further and characterizes the demonstration of trance induction as the engaged consideration upon the proposal or the predominant thought. The fear of a great many people that subliminal specialists will have the option to get into their oblivious and cause them to do and think things outside their ability to control is inconceivable as per the individuals who follow this line of reasoning.

The idea of the mind has additionally been the determinant of the various originations about the recommendation. The individuals who accepted that the reactions given are through the oblivious mind, for example, on account of Milton Erickson, raise the instances of utilizing aberrant recommendations. Huge numbers of these aberrant proposals, for example, stories or representations, will shroud their expected importance to cover it from the cognizant mind of the subject. The subconscious recommendation is a type of hypnosis that depends on the hypothesis of the oblivious mind. If the oblivious mind was not being utilized in hypnosis, this sort of recommendation would not be conceivable. The contrasts between the two gatherings are genuinely simple to perceive; the individuals who accept that the recommendations will go fundamentally to the cognizant mind will utilize direct verbal guidelines and proposals, while the individuals who accept the proposals will go essentially to the oblivious mind will utilize stories and analogies with concealed implications.

In both of these hypotheses of figured, the member should have the option to concentrate on one article or thought. This permits them to be driven toward the path that is required to go into the hypnotic state. When the recommendation stage has been finished effectively, the member will, at that point, have the option to move into the third stage, powerlessness.

Powerlessness

After some time, it has been seen that individuals will respond contrastingly to hypnosis. A few people find that they can fall into a hypnotic stupor reasonably effectively and don't need to invest a lot of energy into the procedure by any means. Others may find that they can get into the hypnotic daze, however, simply after a drawn-out timeframe and with some exertion. Still, others will find that they can't get into the hypnotic stupor, and significantly after proceeding with endeavors, won't arrive at their objectives. One thing that specialists have discovered intriguing about the weakness of various members is that this factor stays steady. If you have had the option to get into a hypnotic perspective effectively, you are probably going to be a similar path for an incredible remainder. Then again, if you have consistently experienced issues in arriving at the hypnotic state and have never been entranced, at that point, almost certainly, you never will.

There have been a few distinct models created after some time to attempt to decide the defenselessness of members to hypnosis. A portion of the more established profundity scales attempted to construe which level of a daze the member was in through the discernible signs that were accessible. These would incorporate things, for example, unconstrained amnesia. A portion of the more present-day scales works to quantify the level of self-assessed or watched responsiveness to the particular recommendation tests that are given, for example, the immediate proposals of unbending arm nature.

As per the examination that has been finished by Deirdre Barrett, there are two kinds of subjects that are considered profoundly vulnerable to the impacts of subliminal therapy. These two gatherings incorporate dissociates and fantasizers. The fantasizers will score high on the assimilation scales, will have the option to effortlessly shut out the boosts of this present reality without the utilization of hypnosis, invest a great deal of their energy wandering off in fantasy land, had fanciful companions when they were a youngster, and experienced childhood in a situation where nonexistent play was energized.

CHAPTER 2:

How to Transform Your Mindset

O ur minds are very strong tools in our lives. How we behave and react to situations is a result of our mental conditioning and thought process. For a person to transform a certain behavior, for instance, quitting smoking or kicking an addiction to electronic devices, the transformation must start in mind first. What we instill in our subconscious minds is want we portray outside. For instance, if you are overweight due to overeating or eating the wrong kinds of foods, there may be underlying issues to your behavior. To transform your behavior, you must begin by transforming your mind. By use of hypnosis, a person can transform their mind and achieve their desired change.

Using Hypnosis to Transform Your Mind

The idea of hypnotherapy brings out reactions ranging from "cross-arm and wary in dismay" to "shocked in unadulterated amazement and surprise." There is no denying the supernatural quality encompassing spellbinding; it stays to puzzle individuals' psyches around the world.

As a result, we tend to live our lives amid a society in which the day to day rush of events doesn't leave us much time for thought and contemplation. This means that we are faced with making difficult choices in terms of dealing with our happiness and wellbeing.

Fortunately, this idea is a long way from a reality of true to life when you grasp spellbinding. In this way, we have a greatly improved idea.

What about utilizing the incredible intensity of hypnotherapy rather than manufacturing a universe of a completely perfect world?

Since there is a persuading reason for hypnotherapy behind the cloak of wizardry and visual impairment, to fix our brains, bodies, and in the long run, our universe.

As a general rule, trance has been utilized worldwide as an instrument for mending for in any event 4,000 years; however, science has just begun to exhume this entrancing riddle in most recent years. Their outcomes hugely affect our ability to change our thoughts and convictions, conduct, and practices, just as our recognition and reality to improve things.

In any case, most importantly, science has discovered a solid reality: entrancing is valid. What's more, on the off chance that you accept you've never had mesmerizing, accept again.

Hypnosis' characterizing practices are:

Increased suggestibility. Making musings progressively open and responsive.

Improved creative thinking. Creation in the eye of our psyches of striking, frequently illusory symbolism.

Without thinking, discernment. Quieting the cognizant systems that create thoughts while improving passionate mindfulness.

These 3 characterizing highlights make spellbinding a particular and effective instrument for private transformation.

A large portion of the issues that unleash destruction on the globe today happen because we have significant mental wounds to which there has been no inclination.

We download information from the globe around us at lightning speed until we're around 9 years of age. During this minute, our subliminal feelings and practices are normally shaped — before we built up our balanced reasoning (got when our mind frames the prefrontal cortex).

In our childhood, for instance, someone can let us know, "you're ugly." At the time, our brains can't defend the likelihood that any individual who reveals to us this will have a poor day or experience the ill effects of their psychological wounds. Rather, our energetic, honest personalities accept, "goodness, I'm frightful." That works for "you're stunning" on a kinder note, just as some other great attestation.

We are important making machines in this incredibly porous minute in our life. We quickly credit importance to them when certain events happen in our youthfulness. What produces our subliminal convictions is that allotted significance.

This is the place hypnotherapy comes in. Nothing fixes these significantly established enthusiastic wounds more rapidly than the hypnotherapy prescription. We have discovered that, in the condition of mesmerizing, we can get to and interface legitimately with these intuitive zones of our psyche—without our normal cognizant reasoning.

During trance, a trance inducer controls their patients back to their youth's zenith occasions. The patient can reassign centrality to them once recollections of the case reach them.

Reprogramming Your Mind through Hypnosis

Your intuitive personality has an enormous impact in dealing with your background—from the sorts of sustenance you eat to the exercises you take each day, the income level you get, and even how you react to unpleasant conditions.

Your intuitive feelings and understandings manage all of it. In a nutshell, your subliminal personality resembles an airplane's auto-pilot work. Following a particular way has been pre-modified, and you cannot go astray from that course except if you initially change the customized guidelines.

The "intuitive" is your mind's part that works underneath your customary arousing cognizance level. At this moment, you are primarily utilizing your cognizant personality to peruse these expressions and retain their centrality. However, your subliminal personality works hectically in the background, engrossing or dismissing information dependent on a present perspective on the globe around you. When you were a tyke, this present observation began to shape. Your intuitive personality drenches like wipe data with each experience.

While you were youthful, your consciousness rejected nothing since you had no prior perspectives that would negate what it saw. It simply recognized that it was genuine every one of the information you acquired during your initial puberty. You can almost certainly observe why this sometime down the road turns into an issue. Each time you were called by somebody stupid, useless, slow, apathetic, or more terrible, your subliminal personality put away the information for reference.

You may likewise have messages about your life potential or requirements relying upon your physical aptitudes, the shade of the skin, sex, or money related status. By the minute you were 7 or 8 years of age, you had a solid premise of religious on all the programming you viewed from people in your lives, network shows, and other natural impacts.

Since you are developed, you may figure you can simply dispose of the destructive or false messages you've consumed in your initial life. However, it isn't so basic. Keep in mind this information is put away underneath your cognizant awareness level. The main minute you understand this is the point at which it constrains your advancement in building up an actual existence that is adjusted, prosperous, and gainful.

Have you, at any point, endeavored to arrive at a target and consistently undermined yourself? Goading, right? It is fundamental to comprehend that regardless of what you do, you are not flawed or destined to come up short. You are bound to have some old, customized messages that contention with the new conditions that you need to make.

This is incredible news since it suggests that on the off chance that you first set aside the effort to reconstruct your intuitive personality, you can achieve pretty much anything! Before we discover how to reconstruct your psyche, it's fundamental to comprehend that the programming proceeds right up 'til today. You draw certain discoveries with each experience you have and store the messages that will direct your future conduct.

Procedures to Reprogram Your Mind

There are numerous particular techniques to overwrite your psyche mind's constrained or hurtful messages.

You could work with every one of these methodologies simultaneously; however, on the off chance that you pick only a couple of procedures to start, it will be significantly more effective. Rather than skipping around and weakening your endeavors, you need to give them complete consideration. Keep in mind; additional strategies can generally be consolidated after some time.

Impacts From the Environment Around You

Have you, at any point, respected your psyche mind's effect on your setting? Keep in mind that your subliminal personality is always engrossing information and reaching determinations dependent on that information and framing convictions.

Envision what sorts of messages are being ingested into your psyche if your day by day condition is loaded up with cynicism and struggle. Your first meditation is to carefully limit from this time on the antagonism to which you are oppressed. Except if you thoroughly need to watch the news and avoid investing a lot of energy with' lethal' people.

Rather, search for helpful information to peruse and watch, and burn through the vast majority of your minute with people who are sure and effective. You will locate that all the more reassuring messages are retained in your brain after some time, which will change how you see yourself and your potential.

Representation

Your subliminal personality responds well to pictures. Representation is an amazing method to utilize ideal, incredible pictures to program your brain. Attempt to picture advantageous scenes that element you and your background for 10–15 minutes every day.

Here are a few things you should envision:

- Fulfilling connections

- Passionate work

- An exquisite home extraordinary excursion

Whatever else you need to bring into your lives. As you do this always, you wind up redrawing the unfavorable pictures put away from your past encounters, concerns, concerns, and questions. Make sure to emanate incredible, positive emotions as you picture these excellent things in your brain to further expand the quality of representation. Permit love, satisfaction, appreciation, and harmony to move through you as though you truly had these encounters.

The message will be consumed by your subliminal personality, as though it were real! This is the genuine excellence of perception—the expert to sidestep confining messages and focuses on wonderful pictures that are altogether retained into your subliminal to replay later.

Affirmations

Affirmations are another effective method to place positive messages into your intuitive.

On the off chance that you observe a couple of straightforward standards, they work best:

- **Positively word them in the current state**. Declare "I'm certain and fruitful" rather than "I will be sure and effective," because are concentrating on a future condition doesn't compute with your intuitive personality — it just comprehends this time. Utilize helpful articulations too. Saying "I am not a disappointment" is determined as "I am a disappointment" since it is incomprehensible for your intuitive to process negative things.

- **Call for the proper feelings**. Saying "I am rich" while feeling poor just sends your subliminal clashing messages. Whatever words you state right now, attempt to feel the sentiments because your intuitive will be bound to think it.

- **Repeat, reiteration, redundancy**. On the off chance that you simply state it on more than one occasion, certifications don't work. Discuss them for the most elevated results ordinarily during the day. The decent thing about this is you can reveal to yourself attestations, so they can accommodate your routine flawlessly.

The Excitement of the Brain Through Binaural Beats

Another regular procedure is to utilize sound chronicles that purposefully change the recurrence of your brainwaves. It might seem like something from a sci-fi film. However, records are overwhelmingly positive from people who have endeavored these sound projects.

Contingent upon what you're doing at any predefined minute, your brainwaves fall into a particular recurrence:

- Gamma when you're engaged with certain motor capacities

- Beta when you're completely mindful and effectively centering

- Alpha when you've loosened up, Theta when you're lazy or languid.

- Delta when you are in significant rest

"Binaural beats" lead when two tones are performed at particular frequencies, causing an unmistakable example in your brainwaves. For example, you tune in to a sound that causes the alpha state if you needed to move from worried to lose. These sound projects can help reconstruct your subliminal personality by building up a progressively responsive gathering for advantageous messages to be introduced.

Research has demonstrated that when you are extremely loose, as in the alpha or theta expresses, your intuitive personality is increasingly open to new information. Utilizing cerebrum preparing sound projects alongside insistences or perception can be a solid blend because your subliminal personality enables its protections to assimilate any message you need to program in promptly.

Simply unwind and focus on good pictures!

CHAPTER 3:

Emotional Eating and How Overcoming Emotional Barriers

What Is Emotional Eating?

People usually eat to beat physical hunger. However, some people are relying on food as a source of comfort or to address their negative emotions. Some also use food as a reward whenever they achieve their goals or when celebrating special events like birthdays or weddings. When you use food as a cover or a solution for extreme emotions, then you suffer from emotional eating. The feelings that trigger your eating are mostly negative, for example, stress, loneliness, sadness, or when you are grieving. However, it is not only the negative emotions that can cause emotional eating; some positive emotions such as happiness or feelings of comfort can also trigger emotional eating.

There is a difference in the way people use food to address their emotions. While some people rely on food when they are in the middle of their life situations, others may find comfort in food soon after the situation is over. They use food as a recovery tool. A problem associated with emotional eating is that it may prevent you from utilizing other adaptive approaches to problems. You should also know that emotional eating does not solve the issues you are going through. If anything, it only serves to make you feel worse. After eating, the original emotional problem remains unsolved, and on top of it, you find yourself feeling guilty about overeating. It is, therefore, essential for you to identify the problem of emotional eating and to take timely appropriate measures to stop it.

How to Recognize Emotional Eating

The best way for you to know if you are suffering from emotional eating is to find out whether you always eat because you are hungry or you eat impulsively. You should pay attention to your emotions and how you usually cope with them. Find out if you are utilizing food just for hunger or you are unconsciously overeating.

Once you are sure you have an emotional eating problem, take appropriate steps to stop it. This is because not all the food you eat is healthy. You will occasionally find yourself eating unhealthy food such as junk food and sweets, which could be detrimental to your health.

Common Features of Emotional Hunger

It is easy for you to mistake emotional hunger for normal physical hunger. You, therefore, need to learn how to make a distinction between the two forms of hunger. The following are some of the hints you can use to tell the difference between the two kinds of hunger:

Emotional Hunger Comes Unexpectedly

You tend to experience emotional hunger suddenly. The feelings of craving will then overwhelm you, forcing you to look for food urgently. On the other hand, feelings of physical hunger tend to grow gradually. Also, when you are physically hungry, you will not be overwhelmed suddenly by hunger, not unless you have gone for days without food.

Emotional Hunger Desires for Some Specific Food

If you are physically hungry, any food is right for you. Physical hunger is not too selective on the type of food to consume. You will feel satisfied eating healthy food like fruits and vegetables. On the other hand, emotional hunger tends to be selective on the food to consume. In most cases, emotional hunger craves unhealthy foods, such as sweets, snacks, and junk food. The craving for these foods tends to be overwhelming and urgent. You may experience strong desires for such food as pizza or cheesecake, and you have no appetite for any other type of food.

Emotional Eating Lacks Concern for Consequences

If you are involved in emotional eating, then in most cases you find yourself eating without any concern about the consequences of overeating on your general wellbeing. You also eat without paying attention to the food you are consuming. You are not concerned about the quality of the food or its nutritional value. All you care about is the quantity of the food to satisfy your craving. Your goal will be to eat as much food as possible. On the other hand, when you are eating because of physical hunger, you will be conscious of the quality and the quantity of food you are consuming. You will be concern about the health benefits of the food you are eating. You will also choose to eat a very well-balanced diet, which will prevent your body from overeating junk foods.

Emotional Hunger Is Insatiable

If you are suffering from emotional eating, your hunger cannot be satisfied no matter the amount of food you have consumed. Hunger as a craving will refuse to get out of your mind. You will keep craving more and more food, and soon, you will find yourself eating continuously without a break. On the other hand, physical hunger is satisfied the moment your stomach is full. You may experience feelings of physical hunger only during specific times of the day. This could be the response of your body once you have conditioned it to receive food at times of the day.

Emotional Hunger Is Located on Your Mind

Unlike physical hunger, the craving for food originates from your mind. Emotional hunger involves the obsession originating from your mind on some specific type of food. You find yourself unable to ignore or overcome this obsession. You then give in to it and reach for your favorite food.

On the other hand, physical hunger originates from the stomach. You feel the hunger pang from your stomach. You can also occasionally feel growling from your belly whenever you are hungry.

Emotional Hunger Comes with Guilt and Regrets

When you are suffering from emotional eating, deep down, you know your eating does not come with any nutritional benefits. You will then have feelings of guilt or even shame. You know you are doing your health a lot of harm, and you may start regretting your actions. On the other hand, physical eating involves eating to satisfy your hunger. You will not suffer any feelings of shame or guilt for meeting your bodily needs.

Causes of Your Emotional Eating

For you to succeed in putting a stop to your emotional eating habits, you need to find out what triggers them. Find out the exact situations, feelings, or places that make you feel like eating whenever you are exposed. Below are some of the common causes of emotional eating:

Stress

One symptom of stress is hunger. You tend to experience the feeling of hunger whenever you are stressed. When you are stressed, your body responds by producing a stress hormone known as Cortisol. When this hormone is produced in high quantities, it will trigger a craving for foods that are salty or sugary in nature as well as any fried food. These are the food which gives you a lot of instant energy and pleasure.

If you do not control stress in your life, you will always be seeking relief in unhealthy food.

Boredom

You could be eating to relieve yourself of boredom. You can also resort to eating to beat idleness. Besides, you may be using food to occupy your time because you do not have much to do. Food can also fill your void and momentarily distract you from the hidden feelings of directionless and dissatisfaction with yourself. Whenever you feel purposeless, you tend to reach out for food to make you feel better. However, the truth is that food can never be a solution to any of your negative emotions.

Childhood Habits

Emotional eating could be a result of your childhood habits. For example, if your parents used to reward your good behaviors with foods such as sweets, ice cream, or pizza, you may have carried these habits to your adulthood. You will find yourself rewarding yourself with your childhood snack whenever you accomplish a given task. You can also be unconsciously eating because of the nostalgic feelings of your childhood. This happens when you always cherish the delicacies you used to eat in your childhood. Food can also serve as a powerful reminder of your most cherished childhood memories, for example, if you were eating cookies with your dad during your outings together. Whenever you miss your dad, your first instinct is to reach out for the cookies.

Social Influences

Occasionally, you may need to go out with your friends and have a good time. During such outings, you can share a meal to relieve stress. However, such social events can lead to overeating. You can find yourself overeating at the nudge of your close friends or family encourages you to go for an extra serving. It is easy to fall into their temptation.

Avoiding Emotions

You may use eating as a way of temporarily avoiding the emotions you are feeling, such as the feeling of anxiety, shame, resentment, or anger. Eating is a perfect way to prevent negative distractions, albeit temporarily.

Habits and Practices, You Can Use to Overcome Emotional Eating to Lose Weight

Practice Healthy Lifestyle Habits

You will handle life's shortcomings better when you are physically strong, happy, and well-rested. However, if you are exhausted, any stressful situation you encounter will trigger the craving for food. In this regard, you need to make physical exercise part of your daily routine. You also need to have enough time to sleep to feel rested. Moreover, engage yourself in social activities with others. Create time for outings with family or close friends.

Practice Mindfulness by Eating Slowly

When you eat to satisfy your feelings rather than your stomach, you tend to eat so fast and mindlessly that you fail to savor the taste or texture of your food. However, when you slow down and take a moment to savor every bite, you will be less likely to indulge in overeating. Slowing down also helps you to enjoy your food better.

Accept All Your Feelings

Emotional eating is often triggered by feelings of helplessness over your emotions. You lack the courage to handle your feelings head-on, so you seek refuge in food. However, you need to be mindful of your feelings. Learn to overcome your emotions by accepting them. Once you do this, you regain the courage to handle any feelings that triggers your emotional eating.

Take a Moment Before Giving in to Your Cravings

Typically, emotional eating is sudden and mindless. It takes you by surprise, and often you may feel powerless in stopping the urge to eat. However, you can control the sudden urges to reach for food if you take a moment of 5 minutes before you give in. This allows you a moment to reconsider your decisions and eventually get the craving out of your mind.

Find Other Alternative Solutions to Your Emotion

Actively look for other solutions to address your feelings other than eating. For example, whenever you feel lonely, instead of eating, reach out for your phone and call that person who always puts a smile on your face. Look for good alternatives to food that you can rely on to feel emotionally fulfilled. If you feel anxious, learn to do exercises.

CHAPTER 4:

Change Bad Eating Habits Through Hypnosis

You realize you need to quit eating; however, you basically can't. You know you've had enough burgers to last you for the following three meals, yet you just can't resist the urge to keep on crunching ceaselessly as though your life relied upon it. You realize that you need to battle it, yet you can't make sense of how to end binge eating. It will be a long stretch; however, the uplifting news is there are ways on the most proficient method to stop binge eating, and these cures are necessarily inside yourself discipline's scope.

Binge or emotional eating is the propensity to the gorge to adapt to negative sentiments or stress; for example, when cutoff times are closer or remaining burden is accumulating as far as possible. Studies point to low self-regard as the most well-known reason for binge eating. Different variables incorporate the absence of help from family or companions, stress, and weight. People with weight issues tend to eat considerably more when they are emotionally upset, and when they start, they get lost about how to end binge eating.

In the USA alone, there are about 1.9 million individuals, or one out of 142 people has a binge eating issue. This sickness rises above sex and age. Step-by-step instructions to end binge eating is, for the most part, about building up the conviction to quit overeating NOW, before other wellbeing confusions begin springing up on you.

There's no compelling reason to feel lost anyway because here are some basic strides on the most proficient method to end binge eating that you can follow.

1. The initial step on the best way to end binge eating is to search for the clinical help of a therapist or a specialist who can capably set up your treatment, an endless supply of turmoil.

2. After seeing your primary care physician, ensure that you adhere to your treatment plan. There are different treatments that experts use with the goal that patients can control their inordinate yearnings for nourishment. Well, known medicines are psychological, social therapy, relational psychotherapy, and the utilization of antidepressants to counter the inclination to indulge in emotional pressure. The specialists are there to control the patient. However, the achievement principally lies on the patient.

3. Uncover those smothered sentiments to the specialist. The propensity for overeating didn't happen medium-term. There may be encounters or injuries that have made you take comfort from nourishment. Closure binge eating might be quicker if the specialist comprehends what these underlying feelings and meetings are, so the individual in question can help you outline good strive after nourishment and emotional learning.

4. Leave your storage room. Since it's a sickness, it is something that you ought not to mind your own business. There are a great many others out there who are having some issues with you are. The most effective method to end implies connecting with whatever care groups are accessible inside your range.

5. Converse with your primary care physician about changing your way of life to return you to good shape of stable living.

The most effective method to end binge eating requires solid self-discipline. Besides, depending on nourishment, you might need to take up different exercises to alleviate you when you are in an emotional session. Attempt yoga and various types of activities, or just connect with a companion or a care group at whatever point the urge comes up.

It has been seen that binge eating is progressively frequent in creating western nations and has been expanding in recent years. That is why you don't need to feel that you are distant from everyone else. There are many different ways that you can turn to the most proficient method to end binge eating. Recollect this is a problematic issue and ought not to be trifled with or be embarrassed about.

Significantly, you begin revamping a stable relationship with yourself to defeat the binge eating issues. It's certainly something that requires some investment to do, but on the other hand, it's the most significant relationship you have, and it must be supported.

Having a stable and positive relationship with yourself is significant. All things considered, how would you part with affection if you can't cherish yourself? If you have a respectable love for yourself, continue doing something that will continuously raise it to another level. A superior level. If you have been binge eating for quite a while and have discovered that your self-love simply isn't there, attempt a portion of these tips to improve the relationship and love for yourself. We ought to never abandon ourselves and on beating binge eating issues.

To manufacture a superior relationship with yourself and discover self-love progressively, attempt these eight hints:

1. Set solid limits. Figure out how to state no when you would prefer not to accomplish something, need more time, or are excessively worried about everything else going on in your life. You need to focus on yourself, and it's significant that you have limits, so the possibility to binge eat isn't as definite.

2. Find a workable pace. At the point when you invest energy alone, you will find such a large number of things about yourself that may have covered up for quite a while.

3. Practice positive self-talk. Negative emotions can outdo you and cause you to feel awful. Envision gorging without beating yourself up. Envision not permitting yourself to have any liable sentiments or self-contempt about the binge. Envision not being at the most reduced level conceivable. Consider what solid self-talk can accomplish for you and the closure of the battle with binge eating issues. Giving up and pushing ahead can genuinely turn your life around!

4. Figure out how to excuse. Absolution is something that can be difficult to do. Now and again, it can appear as though holding resentment bodes well. At the point when you hold resentment, your emotions stifle the development that is required to develop as an individual.

6. Show your feelings. It is anything but a solid plan to hold your opinions in. Instead, it's ideal for letting whatever emotion you are learning about come! Show your displeasure, bliss, or pity. Letting your actual feelings show you will yet be another positive development of not gorging.

7. Be consistent with yourself. Rather than continually beating yourself down, why not begin to laud the beneficial things that are going on in your life? Begin being compatible with yourself by indicating support for new ideas and adulating what you have just practiced.

8. No more flawlessness: Just act naturally. Quit attempting to be a person or thing that you are most certainly not! Show your real nature and be glad for the individual you have become throughout everyday life. Praise who you are by doing whatever it takes not to be great. There's nothing of the sort, and you'll never arrive at that objective. Permit yourself to be you simply!

The Real Issue with Emotional Eating

The issue with emotional eating isn't that we eat in light of feelings. If that were the situation, the arrangement would be as straightforward as finding an interruption in a snapshot of extraordinary sentiments. The thought is that if you occupy yourself, you will abstain from gorging. The center turns into a break rather than managing your feeling.

The main problem with emotional eating is our fear of permitting our feelings a chance to surface. What is so terrifying about feelings? In our quest for having a place and fear of being condemned, we stifle sentiments that we know don't think about what is going on in reality. They appear unexpectedly and don't address us in a natural language that we can react to without much effort. Like a youngster that won't quit annoying until they get what they need, sentiments divert us from keeping an eye on what needs to do. The battle between our feelings and keenness drain us of vitality and take steps to toss us into a wild emotional typhoon. Imagine a scenario where we can't bring ourselves back. What is the benefit of recognizing feelings that would freely humiliate us? We accept that if we acknowledge our sentiments, we would need to follow up on them. Our activities may, for all time, harm our own and expert connections. We would be marked emotional and nonsensical, prompting the most exceedingly awful destiny an individual can persevere estrangement.

So, we control our feelings by returning them where they have a place in our bodies. We conceal our sentiments and continue to act in what we see to be adequate conduct. Our notoriety stays unblemished, and connections endure one more near calamity. Until our bodies make some noise and state "enough." The possibility that feelings are damaging and that the agony is deplorable is the main thrust behind the motivation to stifle our inclination at any expense. Similarly, as we endeavor to occupy a youngster amidst a hissy fit with sweets, we divert ourselves with nourishment.

Consider the possibility that sentiments got middle of the road. Imagine a scenario in which we had confidence that our feelings would vanish as fast as they showed up all alone. Imagine a situation where we regarded feelings as a significant aspect of the human condition. Imagine a situation in which we could simply be with them without blame or disgrace. Would we need an interruption? Would there be a requirement for emotional eating?

Behind the entirety of life's poor decisions is fear. At the point when we surrender to fear and search for self-defensive instruments, we damage our ideal experience of life. We limit our development potential and further harm our self-regard.

Weight loss training works by creating a protected spot where fearlessness and self-certainty are the stages from which decisions are made. When you decide to take part in the chance of permitting yourself to be trained, you will learn procedures that will empower you to grasp your feelings instead of stifling them. By recognizing emotions, you will recover control and praise the totality of what your identity is. You will let loose vitality recently devoured by the inward clash and direct it towards satisfying your fantasies.

CHAPTER 5:

Build a Healthy Relationship with Food

Would it be advisable for you to start a better eating routine or create smart dieting propensities to get in shape? For some individuals, the main thing they consider with regards to weight reduction is that they ought to start eating better. In all actuality, for long-haul benefits, the propensity for eating nutritiously is a vastly improved alternative for a few reasons.

The very notice of "starting a better eating routine" infers that you will later fall off of that diet. That in that spot reveals to you that eating fewer carbs is a momentary way to deal with a way of life issue. Sure, craze diets may work for the time being, yet over the long haul, they, for the most part, don't give any genuine advantage. Individuals need to shed pounds and keep it off. By learning the best possible strategies for weight control and keeping up smart dieting propensities, you are substantially more liable to reach and remain at your ideal weight. Giving exceptionally nutritious foods in the best possible sums is the ideal approach to fuel your body and control your weight.

Many "prevailing fashion eats less" increase momentary fame for the straightforward explanation that they give present moment, quick weight reduction, these eating regimens are frequently founded on taking out some nutritious foods and supplanting them with shakes, caffeinated drinks or other enchantment elixirs, diet pills, high fiber blends or costly prepared dinners. Some of the time, definitely diminishing your calories is a piece of these weight control plans. It is imperative to recollect that your body is powered by the nourishment you eat. So as to work at an elevated level, be solid and enthusiastic, it is indispensable to supply your body with exceptionally nutritious foods. Expelling nutritious foods from your eating regimen in a hurry to get more fit can't insightful choice. At times quick weight reduction can accomplish more mischief than anything.

A great many people comprehend that your body's digestion is imperative to weight control. Think about your digestion as your degree of vitality use. Utilizing less energy can prompt weight gain, since muscle to fat ratio is an abundance vitality that gets put away in fat cells. By diminishing weight too quickly it can really make your body hinder your digestion. This, thus, can make you sleepover weight after the underlying quick weight reduction of an eating routine. Known as the yo-yo impact, this is a main source of disappointment for people hoping to get thinner and keep it off. By joining appropriate dietary patterns and reasonable exercise, you can successfully keep up your digestion working at its legitimate level, which will help with controlling your weight. Muscle-fortifying activity, which straightforwardly expands your digestion, is significant, as is normal cardio aerobic exercise.

A couple of key focuses on appropriate eating ought to be remembered. Eating a few generally little estimated dinners and snacks for the duration of the day is a superior methodology than bigger, less continuous suppers. Try not to skip breakfast - it truly is the most significant dinner of the day. Eating normally keeps up your digestion. Select crisp foods and genuine items, including natural food sources, are vastly improved nourishment decisions than exceptionally handled, substance, and sodium-filled foods.

Numerous individuals believe that eating nutritiously is hard to achieve. The methodology one should take is to create good dieting propensities to get in shape, keep up legitimate weight, and augment your wellbeing. Propensities, both great and awful, are difficult to break. When you set up great dietary patterns, those propensities will be generally simple to keep up for the basic season; your eating techniques are only that - a propensity. Some portion of building up a decent nourishing project is figuring out how to basic food items look for good nourishment decisions. Most visits to the market lead you to similar paths and choosing similar nourishment things. By becoming accustomed to continually purchasing a choice of sound, nutritious foods, it will guarantee that you have these things in your home.

Another misinterpretation about appropriate eating is that nutritious foods are exhausting, tasteless, and not delicious. Nothing can be further from reality. Legitimate nourishment arrangement, cooking techniques, nutritious plans, and sound nourishment substitution can prompt some amazingly solid and delectable dishes.

With the best possible disposition towards your wholesome propensities, it very well may be enjoyment, sound, and scrumptious approach to legitimate weight control. The feared "starting a better eating routine" approach can stay away from as you create smart dieting designs on your approach to great wellbeing and legitimate weight reduction. In the event that you really record what you are eating regularly, you presumably will drop your jaw with sickening apprehension. We never think to include the little tidy portion size piece of candy here and the two treats to really observe the significant effect it is having on our weight control plans. The ideal approach to accomplish a solid way of life, to the extent our weight control plans go, is eating more products of the soil. We as a whole know it, so for what reason do we head for the potato chips aisle in the supermarket rather than the produce segment?

Essentially it comes down to this. Low-quality foods trigger our craving and leave us aching for additional. Ever wonder why eating one minimal honest Cheez-it prompts eating a large portion of a case? One taste triggers your body to need to continue eating. Presently in the event that you could condition yourself to do that with red grapes, we could accomplish that solid way of life. It might be hard to do, however, not feasible. Here are 5 different ways to condition yourself to settle on more beneficial nibble decisions.

Smart Dieting Ha Portions #1: Out of Sight, Out of Mind

On the off chance that you don't have shoddy nourishment in your kitchen, you won't eat it. It truly is that straightforward. I am the sort of individual who needs something to eat while I watch my daily film, and I will, in general, get the terrible stuff. The main occasions I don't is the point at which I cannot. Do your shopping for food directly after you have eaten an enormous supper so you won't be eager for awful foods, yet rather great food sources. Leave the store with no low-quality nourishment yet with plenty of products of the soil. Your satchel and your tummy will thank you over the long haul.

Good Dieting Ha Portions #2: Add Fruits and Vegetables to Your Dishes

Some of the time, it is difficult to plunk down with a couple of strawberries without the chocolate plunge; you desire something terrible. That is the trigger nourishment shouting to you; however, you need not answer. Cut the strawberries up and add them to a bowl of oat. Toss in a couple of blueberries and raisins. Simply make sure to utilize skim milk and keep the sugar in the cabinet. Organic product has enough normal sweetness without anyone else. Consider it characteristic treats.

When was the last time you got amped up for eating carrot and celery sticks without plunging sauce? Likely never, yet that doesn't mean you never will. Add them to a little serving of mixed greens when you need a tidy portion. No, you cannot suffocate it all in greasy blue cheddar dressing.

That is a similar thing as plunge, is it not? A tad of vinaigrette dressing is the thing that your psyche ought to consider.

Good Dieting Ha Portions #3: Make a Compromise

In the event that you are following the American Diet, your palette presently pines for high salt and high-sugar foods. Stopping is never fruitful when it is done immediately. Individuals think they have to stop all the awful stuff at the same time, and afterward 3 days after the fact they wear out and return to negative behavior patterns. Being sound can't pass up the foods you love.

On the off chance that you need pizza, eat a cat with a bowl of natural product serving of mixed greens rather than French fries. In the event that you need Cheeze-Its, eat a bunch with a bunch of grapes rather than a large portion of the cheez-It box. Straightforwardness into it and gradually improve your dietary patterns.

Good Dieting Ha Portions #4: Load up on Liquids

Commonly we mistake strive after thirst. You think you are starving until you drink a decent reviving glass of water. At that point, your stomach feels somewhat fuller, and you have not included more calories in your midsection line. On the off chance that you make sure to drink fluids on a regular basis, you probably get yourself not in any event, thinking you are eager any longer.

So, in light of that, whenever you fear to request an excess of fettuccine Alfredo at your preferred Italian eatery, drink a tall glass of water before you request. You may want to pass that for a pleasant fresh plate of mixed greens with shrimp or chicken.

Smart Dieting Ha Portions #5: Take A Supplement

Once in a while, we get going in our lives and may have the best expectations to eat healthily; however, we cannot generally find solid foods to eat. Most candy machines don't offer carrot and celery sticks, shockingly. One route around this is to take a day by day supplement

EXTREME WEIGHT LOSS HYPNOSIS

that gives all of you the sustenance you would get on the off chance that you ate heaps of products of the soil. This doesn't mean you should take them and keep eating giggles bars throughout the day, as you may have guessed. Garbage is still garbage.

Eating foods grown from the ground may not be something you are utilized to, however simply like whatever else, it takes some becoming accustomed to. Utilize the tips above to make progress simpler, yet don't take on a similar mindset as a con artist. Con artists never succeed, and in the event that it was simple, everybody would stroll around in very good shape. Carrying on with a sound way of life implies settling on solid decisions. The more you do it, the more benefits you will be.

CHAPTER 6:

Program Your Mind to Slim Your Body

Your mind holds the key to your life. You can either let your mind drive you to happiness or malcontent. The good news is that you have the power to reprogram your subconscious mind to lead the life you desire. When you were younger, your mind was a blank slate; it did not have any existing ideas, beliefs, or interpretation of events. Every time someone said something to you, the subconscious absorbed it and stored it away for reference. For example, if you were called fat, worthless, ugly, embarrassing, all that negative information stored away because the mind is always listening and always impartial.

Now that you are older and know better, you believe that it is merely a matter of getting rid of the false notions that your subconscious took hold of in your childhood and youth. It is easier said than done because the subconscious does not respond to the conscious mind. This is because your programming makes decisions for you. Take, for instance; you start a workout routine or a new diet. Your old programming reverts you to your old habits, and you fail miserably at your set goals. This habit can annoy and frustrate you, almost forcing you to abandon the quest for a healthier lifestyle. Before you embark on programming your mind to your slim body, keep in mind that you are already that person that you intend to become. You need to develop the capacity to find them within yourself. To learn how to reprogram your mind successfully, you must:

Make A Decision

Decide on the exact outcome you wish for yourself. With clarity comes the power to shape your subconscious in the new paths to follow. Once you have settled on what you want for yourself at this moment and in the future, you are offering your mind resources toward the fulfillment of your objectives. Write it down.

Let's say you want to be 17-pounds lighter by summer three months away. That is a clear-cut objective which you have set for yourself. Put it down clearly on paper, place it within sight so you can see it as often as possible. Therefore when "external" forces try to sway you to say, indulging or binge eating, you remember that you have set a goal. You have decided to shed seventeen pounds in three months. All of your mental power is aligned to help you accomplish this task.

Commit

Once you have made a clear decision, commit to sticking by it. Commitment means allowing the decision to inform your choices. You may, however, expect to encounter fear. Fear is the biggest threat to success. The fear of failure drives people into giving up on their dreams-not failure itself. Fear can lead to procrastination of your goals, which in turn feed the fear with negative thoughts such as, "I am better off not trying" or "Why should I risk disappointment in case I fail?" These thoughts cause you to feel even worse than you did before. The best solution for fear is facing it.

Failure is not the end of everything; it is a lesson in itself. Access the first trial, everything you did, and how you did it. Examine if there is a way to modify the exercise to alter the result. Therefore, fear should not hold you back from your goals. Your efforts should be coupled with a commitment to a healthier lifestyle, devotion to overcoming the negative thoughts, and above all, commitment to yourself.

Modify Progress

Allow flexibility in your mental capacity. When you have committed to your decision, check the progress to see what is working and what can be amended. Striking a balance between alteration and overhaul can be difficult if you do not have a guide-be it a plan or a mentor or sponsor.

Do not limit yourself to the "It's my way or the highway" mentality. Having a peripheral vision can direct you to alternative possibilities and opportunities in case problems arise during your course. Adjusting your programming to cater to these speed bumps builds your resilience to challenges. Your subconscious develops a winning attitude where failures become lessons, hurdles become catapults, and change becomes inevitable.

Reprogramming Your Mind to Overcome Limitations

To overcome limiting beliefs, you must first acknowledge them and accept them for what they are and the role they have played in your life to this crucial point. The reason it is of significant importance to accept them is that you cannot change what does not exist. These beliefs are repeated to us by society, causing us to relate negatively with ourselves, with food, money, and others. When you realize that these beliefs do not define your worth, you will start to see your true potential and develop self-confidence in your abilities. You will feel free to win at everything you set your mind.

Note Down Your Personal Limiting Beliefs

While getting rid of all your limitations, write down the beliefs that you have had from childhood that simply do not serve your purpose anymore. For example, "I am overweight" or "I do not look as good as my petite friends." Such beliefs have likely caused you to look upon yourself with disdain. The negative "I am" thoughts are not honestly what you think of yourself unless someone said them to you.

Understand Causality

The circumstances you find yourself in are not the cause of your limiting beliefs, but the effect. Let us take an example of struggling with weight; the reason you are "struggling" is because of your limiting beliefs about food and yourself. Knowing this, you can alter your mentality about your limitations and flip them to work for you instead of against you.

Along with learning how to reprogram our mind, it is essential to note that the subconscious is still taking in new information and using it for reference for future decisions. There are several ways to reprogram your mind successfully.

Change Your Environment

The environment that surrounds us impresses significantly on our minds. Imagine if you always have people talking down at you at work or school. That kind of negativity can lead to a host of psychological problems, including depression.

Remove yourself from toxic environments; the instance you start to notice a pattern of ill-intentioned thoughts. Immerse yourself in an environment that fosters loving and positive thoughts. This way, your mind will absorb all the kind thoughts and gradually begin to reprogram your thought pattern. Support groups are an excellent environment to immerse yourself in because not only are these people working with the same set of circumstances, but some have also succeeded in daily progress. They know how rough it can be; therefore, they are the best reference for guidance and support.

Visualization

Visualization is a powerful reprogramming tool. Try to envision your transformed self in day-to-day activities. Envision your perfect romantic life, professional life, family relationships, financial relationships, as well as how you relate to yourself. See yourself as you would like to lead your life and allow yourself to feel fulfilled in these visions.

When these images are accompanied by emotions of accomplishment, gratitude, and joy, the more effectively they will redraw on your previous images. Your subconscious will see these images as the truth and will guide your decisions based on the repetitive visualization of the images.

For creative visualization to work, you must first change the underlying negative beliefs. This is because the subconscious, being the autopilot, corrects the shift in course whenever you seem to deviate from the norm. Ignoring the limiting beliefs can, by all means, curtail your efforts at reaching your objectives. Address the underlying cause first, or use the mental by-product focus method to attain what you want. This method allows you to focus on something that you do not have negative thoughts about, and therefore, by association helps you achieve what you desire. For example, you may want to travel abroad for summer vacation. You have been saving up for this trip, and you are looking forward to it. Visualizing your perfect self in your ideal trip will enable you to take the necessary steps to shred the undesired 17-pounds.

Help of Affirmations

Affirmations are necessary when you want to focus on another thought pattern. During affirmations, you phrase your statements positively, attach personal meaning to them, and repeat them to yourself multiple times throughout the day. Corresponding emotion helps the subconscious to understand the statements and believe them as the new status quo.

At first, getting your conscious mind on board with affirmations that may seem far-fetched can be difficult. As time goes on, however, the power of these affirmations has taken root into your subconscious, and you start to believe them to be true even with your rational mind.

Fake It Until You Make It

This method builds your self-esteem. It works in the same manner as affirmations but uses actions instead of thoughts and words. While your conscious mind is busy judging you about your deceiving mannerisms, your subconscious is loyally picking up on all the subtle differences in thought and sensation as you fake your way to your desired objective.

Actively changing your behaviors causes a change in habits, and sooner or later, your entire narrative will change.

Help of Hypnosis

Hypnosis is another tool used to reprogram the mind where the hypnotherapist puts you in a state of complete relaxation and reaches into the subconscious mind. Afterward, messages of empowerment and self-reliance are delivered repetitively to the listener. Hypnosis is used to reprogram the self-defeating habits and thoughts that keep you from achieving your goals.

This technique uses creative metaphors, illustrations, and suggestions to rewire the brain. In the wake of hypnosis weight loss studies, women who participated in hypnosis lost twice as much weight as the women who merely watched what they ate. The research, however, is not enough to be conclusive.

The best way to effect hypnosis is to play the messages when you are retiring for the day. As you are about to fall asleep, play the hypnosis tape, and let it carry your mind forward. Doing this in your sleep is more effective because there are limited to no distractions of the conscious mind chatter. The subconscious, being the sponge, absorbs the new thought patterns and rewrites the societal limitations previously held.

All these modes of rewiring your mind are dominant, but how exactly do you know what to expect? What signs do you look for to show improvement before you start discouraging yourself with negative thoughts? In short, when a paradigm shift takes place in your subconscious, you begin to feel a sense of change in your inner and outer self.

Training your mind is much more efficient than using mere willpower to weight loss. Only by repetitive insertion of positivity into the subconscious can new thoughts and habits become ingrained and manifest on the conscious level. To program your mind to become slimmer is not only about combating the eating habits but a general lifestyle approach that focuses on a healthier life that traverses beyond weight.

CHAPTER 7:

Weight Loss Meditation

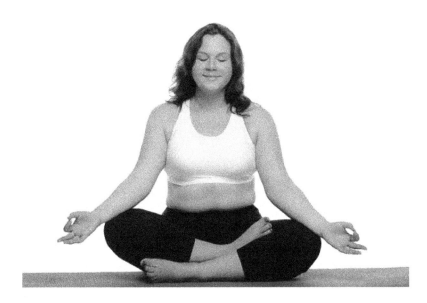

A s we all know, meditation requires sitting still or even lying still. It doesn't sound like the sort of 'exercise' that'll help us lose weight, does it? How can meditation help you lose weight? Astonishing as it may be, weight loss meditation - in particular, 'meaningful meditation' - is increasingly being used by people who want to control the cravings of food and manage overeating. Often, diligent therapy may be used to reduce stress, thereby avoiding the 'comfort eating' arising out of stress. As we become more aware, we become more mindful of our cravings and can learn to pay attention to their underlying emotions, i.e., we can make a more informed decision before simply reaching for that sinful chocolate bar! When you continue feeding conscientiously every day so you will learn to like your food more over time, you'll now be more able to tell when you're full-meaning you'll continue eating fewer calories, of course. It has also been shown that consistent practice of mindful meditation lowers the stress hormone cortical. This is excellent news because high levels of cortical can cause pre-diabetes and central obesity (related to heart disease). In fact, cortical begins a process in our brains that can also lead to elevated hunger and intense cravings.

Don't Multi-Task

Experts say multi-tasking is our biggest enemy of weight control. When practicing careful weight loss meditation, it is important to concentrate on the food and the food alone. A recent study published in the 'Psychological Research' newspaper found that people who watched television at dinner were more likely to over-eat because they found the meal boring.

How Does Meditation Help You Get Weight Loss?

The truth is meditation rewires your consciousness. Feeding consciously is the opposite of feeding mindlessly. Eating more slowly helps your stomach realize when it's full-sometimes the stomach can take up to twenty minutes to signal to the brain that it's full and you shouldn't be hungry anymore. When consuming a limited amount of food, you would actually consume fewer calories all day long, resulting in a healthy and stable weight loss. There are books and CDs available which can teach you meditation techniques to reduce the urge to eat compulsively. Such training guides will help you overcome the cycle of compulsive eating so you can stick to your diet no matter what stress-causing incidents occur in your life. If it takes you a while to see results, don't be discouraged. It can take quite a bit of time to retrain your mind, so you no longer feel the temptation to overeat or eat mindlessly, particularly if it has been a lifelong problem. If you are not getting the effects you expect from directed therapy after giving it a period of time, consider consulting a counselor who is skilled in correcting compulsive behavior. Breaking the stress-based eating process is vital for your ability to stay on a diet and keep weight off after you leave the diet as you will no longer respond to stress by consuming large amounts of calories in your lifetime.

Weight Reduction Hypnosis and Self-Hypnosis

The notion of weight loss using self-hypnosis is definitely fascinating and one that would be nice to believe in. Hypnosis and self-hypnosis are now being used for various purposes, and the theory is embraced by many as much as possible. Strictly speaking, nobody is saying that by hypnosis, as if by a miracle, you can't make pounds go down. No, hypnosis is intended to reprogram your subconscious mind, so you have different behaviors. After all, your actions have much to do with your weight, as well as many other physical health aspects. It doesn't seem so hard to believe.

"Hypnosis" is a relatively new word, coined in the 19th century on the basis of a man named Franz Mesmer (from whom we got the word "mesmerism," meaning basically the same as hypnosis). It means going into a highly suggestible trance state. In more modern years, scientists have established different waves of the brain that exist during those phases. Hypnosis was initially identified with stage hypnotists and magicians, who under hypnosis can induce people to do funny or weird stuff. However, it was also used for therapeutic purposes at the same time. It fits well with the emerging field of psychology, which stressed the subconscious mind's role in our behavior.

Using Weight Loss Hypnosis

If you were using hypnosis to lose weight, how would you go about it? Well, you might get to visit a qualified hypnotherapist. Compared to any type of traditional therapy, this would not be cheap, but it has the advantage of being fast-acting. Many hypnotherapists rely on showing you methods that you can do on your own, and you don't need to go back to them for appointments all the time. A further option is to consider one of the endless videos which will help you lose weight. These can be played at your leisure, but you are unable to play them while driving or doing anything where you need your full conscious attention. Since hypnosis's focus is on the mind, it is also up to you to discover the specific methods that function best. In other terms, you can do your research and find a healthy diet that suits your body (not all person diet works well).

The real aim of weight loss hypnosis is to enable you to do the things you need to do to lose weight without having to exert so much power of will. If your subconscious mind is more aligned with your conscious goals, there is less chance of you sabotaging yourself by cheating on your diet or dropping off your exercise program. It may sound strange or exotic to use hypnosis to lose weight, but it is really just another way to use your mind in a way that supports your goals. Perhaps not for all, but if the idea sounds appealing or at least interesting, you may want to look into some of the weight-loss possibilities of using hypnosis.

CHAPTER 8:

Self-Improvement with Hypnosis

Hypnosis is rewiring your brain to add or to change your daily routine starting from your basic instincts. This happens due to the fact that while you are in a hypnotic state you are more susceptible to suggestions by the person who put you in this state. In the case of self-hypnosis, the person who made you enter the trance of hypnotism is yourself. Thus, the only person who can give you suggestions that can change your attitude in this method is you and you alone.

Again, you must forget the misconception that hypnosis is like sleeping, because if it is, then it would be impossible to give autosuggestions to yourself. Try to think about it like being in a very vivid daydream where you are capable of controlling every aspect of the situation you are in. This gives you the ability to change anything that may bother and hinder you from achieving the best possible result. If you are able to pull it off properly, then the possibility of improving yourself after a constant practice of the method will just be a few steps away.

Career

People say that motivation is the key to improving your career. But no matter how you love your career, you must admit that there are aspects of your work that you really do not like doing. Even if it is a fact that you are good at the other tasks, there is that one duty that you dread. And every time you encounter this specific chore you seem to be slowed down and thus lessening your productivity at work. This is where self-hypnosis comes into play.

The first thing you need to do is find that task you do not like. In some cases there might be multiple of them depending on your personality and how you feel about your job. Now, try to look at why you do not like that task and do simple research on how to make the job a lot simpler. You can then start conditioning yourself to use the simple method every time you do the job.

After you are able to condition your state of mind to do the task, each time you encounter it will become the trigger for your trance and thus giving you the ability to perform it better. You will not be able to tell the difference since you will not mind it at all. However, your coworkers and superiors will definitely notice the change in your work style and in your productivity.

Family

It is easy to improve in a career. But to improve your relationship with your family can be a little trickier. Yet, self-hypnosis can still reprogram you to interact with your family members better by modifying how you react to the way they act. You will have the ability to adjust your way of thinking, depending on the situation. This then allows you to respond in the most positive way possible, no matter how dreadful the scenario may be. If you are in a fight with your husband/wife, for example, the normal reaction is to flare up and face fire with fire. The problem with this approach is it usually engulfs the entire relationship, which might eventually lead up to separation. Being in a hypnotic state in this instance then can help you think clearly and change the impulse of saying words without thinking them through. Anger will still be there, of course, that is the healthy way. But anger now under self-hypnosis can be channeled and stop being a raging inferno. You can turn it into a steady bonfire that can help you and your partner find common ground for whatever issue you are facing. The same applies with dealing with siblings or children. If you are able to condition your mind to think more rationally or to get into the perspective of others, then you can have better family/friends' relationships.

Health and Physical Activities

Losing weight can be the most common reason why people will use self-hypnosis in terms of health and physical activities. But this is just one part of it. Self-hypnosis can give you a lot more to improve this aspect of your life. It works the same way while working out.

Most people tend to give up their exercise program due to the exhaustion they think they can no longer take. But through self-hypnosis, you will be able to tell yourself that the exhaustion is lessened and thus allowing you to finish the entire routine. Keep in mind that your mind must never be conditioned to forget exhaustion, it must only not mind it until the end of the exercise. Forgetting it completely might lead you to not stopping to work out until your energy is depleted. It becomes counterproductive in this case.

Having a healthy diet can also be influenced by self-hypnosis. Conditioning your mind to avoid unhealthy food can be done. Thus, hypnosis will be triggered each you are tempted to eat a meal you are conditioned to consider as unhealthy. Your eating habit can change to benefit you to improve your overall health.

Mental, Emotional and Spiritual Needs

Since self-hypnosis deals directly with how you think, it is then no secret that it can greatly improve your mental, emotional and spiritual needs. A clear mind can give your brain the ability to have more rational thoughts. Rationality then leads to better decision making and easy absorption and retention of information you might need to improve your mental capacity. However, you must set your expectations; this does not work like magic that can turn you into a genius. The process takes time, depending on how far you want to go, how much you want to achieve. Thus, the effects will only be limited by how much you are able to condition your mind.

In terms of emotional needs, self-hypnosis cannot make you feel differently in certain situations. But it can condition you to take in each scenario a little lighter and make you deal with them better. Others think that getting rid of emotion can be the best course of action if you are truly able to rewire your brain. But they seem to forget that even though rational thinking is often influenced negatively by emotion, it is still necessary for you to decide on things basing on the common ethics and aesthetics of the real world. Self-hypnosis then can channel your emotion to work in a more positive way in terms of decision making and dealing with emotional hurdles and problems.

Spiritual need on the other hand is far easier to influence when it comes to doing self-hypnosis. As a matter of fact, most people with spiritual beliefs are able to do self-hypnosis each time they practice what they believe in. A deep prayer, for instance, is a way to self-hypnotize yourself to enter the trance to feel closer to a Divine existence. Chanting and meditation made by other religions also lead and have the same goal. Even the songs during a mass or praise and worship triggers self-hypnosis depending if the person allows them to do so.

Still, the improvements can only be achieved if you condition yourself that you are ready to accept them. The willingness to put an effort must also be there. Effortless hypnosis will only create the illusion that you are improving and thus will not give you the satisfaction of achieving your goal in reality.

How Hypnosis Can Help Resolve Childhood Issues

Another issue that hypnosis can help is those problems from our past. If you have had traumatic situations from your childhood days, then you may have issues in all areas of your adult life. Unresolved issues from your past can lead to anxiety and depression in your later years. Childhood trauma is dangerous because it can alter many things in the brain, both psychologically and chemically.

The most vital thing to remember about trauma from your childhood is that given a harmless and caring environment in which the child's vital needs for physical safety, importance, emotional security, and attention are met, the damage that trauma and abuse cause can be eased and relieved. Safe and dependable relationships are also a dynamic component in healing the effects of childhood trauma in adulthood and make an atmosphere in which the brain can safely start the process of recovery.

Pure Hypnoanalysis is the lone most effective method of treatment available in the world today for the resolution of phobias, anxiety, depression, fears, psychological and emotional problems/symptoms, and eating disorders. It is a highly advanced form of Hypnoanalysis (referred to as analytical hypnotherapy or hypnoanalysis). Hypnoanalysis, in its numerous forms, is practiced all over the world; this method of hypnotherapy can completely resolve the foundation of anxieties in the unconscious mind, leaving the individual free of their symptoms for life.

There is a deeper realism active at all times around us and inside us. This reality commands that we must come to this world to find happiness, and every so often that our inner child stands in our way. This is by no means intentional; however, it desires to reconcile wounds from the past or address damaging philosophies that were troubling to us as children.

So, to disengage the issues that upset us from earlier in our lives we have to find a way to bond with our internal child, we then need to assist in rebuilding this part of us, which in turn will help us to be rid of all that has been hindering us from moving on.

Connecting with your inner child may seem like something that may be hard or impossible to do especially since they may be a part that has long been buried. It is a fairly easy exercise to do and can even be done right now. You will need about 20 minutes to complete this exercise.

Here's what you do: find a quiet spot where you won't be disturbed and find a picture of you as a child if you think it may help.

Breathe in and loosen your clothing if you have to. Inhale deeply into your abdomen and exhale, repeat until you feel yourself getting relaxed; you may close your eyes and focus on getting less tense. Feel your forehead and head relax, let your face become relaxed, and relax your shoulders. Allow your body to be limp and loose while you breathe slowly. Keep breathing slowly as you let your entire tension float away.

Now slowly count from 10-0 in your mind and try to think of a place from your childhood. The image doesn't have to be crystal clear right now, but try to focus on exactly how you remember it and keep that image in mind. Imagine yourself as a child and imagine observing younger you; think about your clothes, expression, hair, etc. In your mind go and meet yourself, introduce yourself to you.

CHAPTER 9:

The Power of Visualization

Continual visualization directs your actions to reflect that of your mental image. This is why it is possible to acquire new skills with creative visualization. You can also use it to give yourself a new set of belief system. You only need to visualize yourself believing in the mental image you create without allowing any resistance into your visualization. You have to reprogram any negative and limiting beliefs if you are to achieve your goal. There are two main ways you can apply this kind of visualization in your life:

• Ensuring a healthy life and banishing bad habits

• Fostering strong relationships

• Manifesting financial abundance

Healthy Living and Banishing Bad Habits

Bad habits often start innocently; an overindulgence during a holiday season that you do not seem to break even when the holidays are over, perfectly normal social situations that slowly get you hooked to the bad behavior, peer pressure, or unhealthy lifestyles. It may be drinking, smoking, over-eating, drug abuse, or gambling. These are all bad habits that undermine any idea you have of making your body and mind healthy. However, to have and maintain a healthy mind you need to have a healthy and happy body.

a) Use Creative Visualization to Heal

The best you can do for yourself is to use creative visualization. With the help of visualization, it is easy to break off any bad habits in your life and acquire the kind of perfect and healthy life you have been dreaming of. Creative visualization can help you quit smoking, reduce drinking and eating, and return your body to better shape in no time.

Through creative visualization, a positive attitude towards improving health can easily be developed. You only need to imagine yourself in that perfect body and health you dream of, and you can easily make it into reality. According to researchers, they found out that an ill person is likely to change the situation by mentally picturing themselves combating their illness. Such action has been proven to reduce the severity of symptoms in a patient and improve their quality and length of life.

However, always remember that when it comes to treating your illness with creative visualization, you must use it with tested procedures and medicines. It is good to get the best professional care and advice to be able to take care of your medical problems fast and effectively. The power of creative thinking only hastens your recovery and enhances the effectiveness of conventional medicine and professional help. It increases your defense for battling any illness you may have.

The whole process of visualizing your well-being is a partnership between you, your doctor, and your body. It is the doctor who determines what is ailing you and begins the medical treatment process to heal your condition. It is up to you to take the information you get from your doctor on where the problem is and pass it to your body. Through creative visualization you get your body to work on the problem at the same time you are receiving conventional medication. This is a process that can easily help you combat any serious and minor illness you have. It involves adopting a positive outlook on your health to keep your immune system in top shape.

b) Use Creative Visualization to Build Strong Core Muscles

As you grow older, your muscles weaken, especially if you are not active. A sedentary life makes your joints calcify, and this often leads to osteoarthritis. When you are young and active, you may not think about the aches and pain of joint problems. However, when you get to your middle ages, these pains become more pronounced. What you need to do is to keep your muscles in good condition.

When using creative visualization, remember that it is impossible to build muscles simply by visualizing them. You need to get active if you want to develop your core muscles and be physically fit. Visualization helps to hasten the process and give you the motivation to keep your mind on the desired results and maintain it.

The benefits of toughening your core muscles can be realized through:

• Improved posture and less low back pain

• Toned muscles that prevent the occurrence of back injuries

• Enhanced physical performance

• Less muscle aches

• Better balance made possible by having lengthened legs

According to physiotherapists and Pilates, the kind of physical and visualization exercise you engage in should emphasize to your body and unconscious mind the importance of keeping your muscles strong and fit to benefit you in all of the above-mentioned areas. They believe that this technique is the key to developing core stability. This is where your abdominal wall, lower back, diaphragm, and pelvis are able to stabilize your body during movement.

How to Combine Physical Exercise with Creative Visualization

Step 1: Do abdominal bracing in a sitting position - Sit up in an alert and straight manner. While maintaining a steady breath, try pulling your navel inwards to touch your spine. It is not enough to imagine this procedure. You must carry it out.

Step 2: Channel energy to your muscles - As you hold your navel in, feel the muscles that are being employed in the process. While in this position and state of mind, visualize yourself directing energy into your muscles from within you.

Step 3: Hold the position - If you are a beginner, you can hold this position for a minimum of 30 seconds. However, the recommended time is five minutes. Always remember to keep breathing evenly.

As you continue with this exercise, you need to try to apply feelings of power, vibrant health, and motivation to your body. This makes it easy to get the inspiration to match your visualization to your physical workouts. However, this is a technique that only works for small toning cases. For an overall toning of your body muscles, you need proper exercising techniques you can combine with creative visualization. Furthermore, if you have an existing health problem, have your doctor check you up and get the relevant professional medication your body requires before you begin this exercise program.

c) Use Creative Visualization to Look After Your Heart

There are very many benefits you get when your heart is healthy. When you ensure your heart is in good condition, you increase your blood flow and the distribution of oxygen all through your body. This lets you enjoy:

• High energy levels and increased endurance

• Low blood pressure

• Reduced body fat and a healthier body weight

• Less stress, anxiety, and depression

• Better sleep

The best way to look after your heart is to engage in aerobics. This is an exercise that causes you to breathe deeply and makes you sweat for a minimum of 20 minutes. Whether it is fast walking, swimming, jogging, biking, or even cross-country skiing, you should be in a position to make a conversation.

How to Combine Aerobics with Creative Visualization

Step 1: Visualize your exercise activity – In your mind, visualize taking a 20-minute jog, fast walk or any other aerobic activity. You can visualize yourself wearing the right exercising clothes and suitable running shoes.

Step 2: Visualize yourself doing the activity – Here, you need to visualize how you feel in the training wear, how the running shoes fit your feet perfectly, the country lane or suburbs in which you are running through, and start the exercise. Feel the power and strength in your feet and envision your arms moving back and forth to the rhythm of your legs. Feel the strength in your body and maintain your balance in a relaxed and simple position.

Step 3: Visualize yourself keeping pace for 20 minutes – In your mind's eye you can make yourself realize that although you are getting tired, you are also energized and can well keep your pace until you are done. Imagine sweat building on your brow; you mop it away; your body feels supple and is moving easily to the finish line.

Step 4: Imagine the scenery – As you jog, imagine passing trees, houses, and you nod to people or wave at them. You should seem to enjoy the fact that they see you serious about your health. In your mind, breath in and out, feel the refreshing coolness of the cool air and how refreshing it is to your lungs.

Step 5: Finish your exercise – You should continue your visualization exercise until you see yourself finish it. See yourself slowing down and returning to a normal walking pace and how your body feels fit and healthy.

While this visualization is still fresh in your mind, plan to get yourself a jogging gear to do a 20 minutes aerobic exercise. After your first jog, you will realize it is easy if you visualize the whole process and act it out as you exercise. You can do this exercise three times a week or more if you can to maintain a healthy heart. Remember to consult your doctor if you have any health issues before you start any aerobic exercises. Additionally, if you feel the exercise is painful for you or you become short of breath, you should stop.

d) Use Creative Visualization to Build Stamina

For you to overcome all the challenges that come with changing bad habits, you need to have both mental and physical stamina. This keeps you going and provides you with the energy you need to overcome through the long haul. Your mental stamina helps you stick to your plans up to their completion. It is the physical stamina that provides you the energy you need to move your body through the whole process of your plans.

When using creative visualization to build your stamina, you need breathing exercises. These exercises not only help you increase your stamina but also provide your body with the endurance you need to complete any activity you are engaged in. With the Chi breathing exercise, your goal should be to relax your shoulders and chest by breathing deeply from within your abdomen.

• Hold your hands over your lower stomach and sit in an upright position

• Breathe deeply until you cannot draw in more air and then let it all out to the last gasp

• Repeat this action more than once

• Visualize yourself breathing in with your hands sucking the air down all the way to your torso and into them

• Visualize yourself exhaling with your hands pushing air back through your stomach

• Slowly take your time settling into a slow, steady, and comfortable rhythm

• Imagine the deep and continuing energy each breath you take brings to you

As you breathe in and out, you should feel your abdomen expanding and contracting and the breathing moving all the way to your pelvic area. Practicing this exercise regularly is a good way to increase your endurance energy levels and build on your stamina level.

CHAPTER 10:

What is Gastric Band Hypnosis

What Is a Gastric Band?

A gastric band is a silicone device that is commonly used to treat obesity.

The device is usually placed on the upper part of the stomach to decrease the amount of food you eat. While on the upper part of the stomach, the band makes a relatively smaller pouch that fills up quickly and slows the consumption rate.

The band works when you make healthy food options, reduce appetite, and limit food intake and volume.

You do not need to experience these challenges when there is a simple and less invasive approach to achieve the same results as in a surgical gastric band.

Hypnotic Gastric Band

It is a natural healthy eating tool that can help control your appetite and your portion sizes. In this sense, hypnosis plays a significant role in helping you lose weight without the risk that comes with surgery.

It is now in the public domain that dieting does not solve lifestyle challenges that require weight loss and management.

Temporary diet plans are less productive, while continuous methods are challenging to maintain. Notably, these plans deprive you of your favorite foods and are too restrictive.

Deep down, you may have a problem with your body weight, and perhaps diets have not worked for you so far.

If you wish to try something that will provide a definite edge, you need to control your cravings for food hypnotically. By reaching this point, it is clear that you have prepared to try hypnosis, which has proven results in aiding weight loss.

How Does Hypnotic Gastric Band Work?

Typically, the conscious mind is not as receptive to suggestions, for it frequently analyzes and critiques them.

Chiefly, the complex network in your brain has different interpretations of the world around you, and most probably, unhelpful and harmful thoughts may have worked their way into that network.

As a result, you automatically become susceptible to uncontrolled unconscious urges such as overeating and ignoring serious bodyweight concerns. The hypnotic gastric band helps you dampen and overcome these uncontrolled thoughts and believe in suggestions that play a significant role in helping you alter your behavior.

Powerful affirmations: A change in lifestyle is mandatory if you wish to have permanent weight loss or control. Powerful statements are vital in changing your lifestyle slowly and surely.

Therefore, you should diligently practice regular affirmations for weight loss to realize the dream of losing weight. Notably, weight control is a direct function of your lifestyle as you are solely responsible for your behavior. In other words, your weight is determined by your mental attitude, the rest you take, physical exertion, and manner and frequency of eating. Use effective weight loss affirmations as a way to initiate the measure from your mind.

For real, it is necessary to change your thinking; otherwise, no form of dieting will ever help. Weight loss affirmations are significant in your mind, for they make you feel comfortable in your desired weight.

You should also consider the affirmations' wording to ensure that you focus on the solution but not the problem. For instance, you should not say, "I am not that fat," for that is the problem. Instead, you should focus on the solution and include words such as "I am getting slimmer" or "I am losing weight daily."

Write down healthy weight affirmations or take a cue from the samples I will provide. Repeating them shows that you are determined and sure to take the bold step of living and looking at a fitter life.

I weigh _ pounds: This affirmation sets the desired weight in your mind, and as you repeat the words, you remind yourself about your destiny and measures that you need to take.

I will achieve the ideal weight to enhance my physical fitness: You embrace lighter weight and improve on physical activity.

I love healthy food, for they help me attain an ideal weight: It promotes healthy eating and craving for healthy food.

I ease digestion by chewing all the food properly to reach my ideal weight: The affirmation is perfect before every meal as it guides the rate and amount of consumption.

I control my weight through a combination of healthy eating and controlling my appetite and my portion sizes:

It is a good idea to repeat these affirmations, among others, especially in front of a mirror, to keep reminding your subconscious mind about your goals. Most importantly, these affirmations work best while meditating or in a trance state. This combination will do wonders in your weight loss endeavor.

Powerful Visualization: With a hypnotic gastric band, your imagination should control your subconscious mind and body as a whole.

Visualizing weight loss means making the image of how you want to be in your mind's eye. It is an excellent tool that triggers the subconscious mind to shape your body to match your mental image. If you visualize accordingly, you will achieve weight loss, improve how you look, and become more energetic. Notably, emotions and thoughts affect the body for better or for worse. Negative thinking, anger, fear, stress, and worry, hurt the body and lead to the production of toxins that adversely affect you. On the other hand, if you are happy, confident, and positive, you energize and strengthen the body.

Learning how to use your subconscious mind in visualization effectively is to your advantage. Besides, it is a mental diet that you should incorporate into your weight loss plan. Chiefly, the success of the hypnotic gastric band will be higher if you eat healthily in addition to affirmations and visualization.

Visualization is such a great tool in the journey of leaving overeating and emotional eating behind. The significance of display lies not in our physical body but in the feeling of overcoming obsessions and challenges with food, weight, perfect body or plagues, and restrictions that keep you on the dieting merry go round.

With the hypnotic gastric band, visualization is a simple process, and you can use these few tips for weight loss.

· Find frequent moments where you sit down for several minutes and quietly visualize your slim body. Ignore all doubts, worries, and negative thoughts and maintain focus on the image.

EXTREME WEIGHT LOSS HYPNOSIS

· Forget your current look and imagine a beautiful and slim you with the ideal weight. See how gorgeous you look in a swimming suit and tight clothing that you always want to wear.

· Visualize peers and family complimenting your slim body and looks. Just watch the whole scene as if it is real and happening now.

· Feel free to construct different versions of these instances or other physical roles, such as dancing or swimming. Visualize yourself hearing compliments from other people about your slim body and watch them as they admiringly glare at you.

· Make the images you create in your mind colorful, realistic, and alive. See yourself in each of these real and exciting scenes in the ideal weight.

Avoid words that may destroy the efforts you may have made and let only the thoughts of your ideal weight and shape into your mind. Powerful visualization works wonders when practiced in hypnosis, for it makes the mental image a possible reality.

CHAPTER 11:

How to Know if
Gastric Band Hypnosis Works for You

H ypnotherapy for weight loss, particularly for portion control, is great because it allows you to focus on creating a healthier version of yourself safely.

When gastric band fitted surgery gets recommended to people, usually because diets, weight loss supplements, and workout routines don't seem to work for them, they may become skeptical about getting the surgery done.

Nobody wants to undergo unnecessary surgery, and you shouldn't have to either. Just because you struggle to stick to a diet, workout routine, or lack motivation does not mean that an extreme procedure like surgery is the only option. In fact, thinking that it is the only option you have left, is crazy.

Some hypnotherapists suggest that diets don't work at all. Well, if you're motivated and find it easy to stick to a diet plan and workout routine, then you should be fine. However, if you're suffering from obesity or overweight and don't have the necessary drive and motivation needed, then you're likely to fail. When people find the courage and determination to recognize that they need to lose weight or actually push themselves to do it, but continuously fail, that's when they tend to give up.

Gastric band hypnotherapy uses relaxation techniques, which are designed to alter your way of thinking about the weight you need to lose, provides you a foundation to stand on and reach your goals, and also constantly reminds you of why you're indeed doing what you're doing. It is necessary to develop your way of thinking past where you're at in this current moment and evolve far beyond your expectations.

Diets are also more focused on temporary lifestyle changes rather than permanent and sustainable ones, which is why it isn't considered realistic at all. Unless you change your mind, you will always remain in a rut that involves first losing and then possibly gaining weight back repeatedly. Some may even throw in the towel completely.

Hypnotherapy for Different Types of Gastric Banding Types of Surgeries

There are three types of gastric banding surgeries that could be used during hypnotherapy. These include:

• Sleeve Gastrectomy

• Vertical Banded Gastroplasty

• Mixed Surgery (Restrictive and Malabsorptive)

Gastric banding surgeries are used for weight loss. Depending on what your goal is with this weight-loss method, you can choose which option works best for you. The great thing about hypnotherapy with gastric band firming surgery is that you can get similar results if you practice the session consistently.

During gastric banding surgery, the surgeon uses a laparoscopy technique that involves making small cuts in the stomach to place a silicone band around the top part of your stomach. This band is adjustable, leaving the stomach to form a pouch with an inch-wide outlet. After you've been banded in surgery your stomach can only hold one ounce of food at a time, which prevents you from eating more than you need to in one sitting. It also prevents you from getting hungry.

Given that it is an invasive procedure, most people don't opt for it as an option to lose weight. During the procedure, you are also placed under anesthesia, which always involves some risks. Nevertheless, the procedure has resulted in up to 45% of excess weight loss, which means that it can work for anyone looking to shed weight they are struggling to lose. The procedure can also be reversed should the patient not be happy with the effects thereof. When reversed, the stomach will return to the initial size it had before the surgery. (WebMD, n.d.)

Undergoing one of these three gastric banding surgeries, there are some side-effects involved, which include the risk of death. However, this is only found in one of every 3000 patients. Other than that, common problems post-surgery include nausea and vomiting, which can be reduced by simply having a surgeon adjust the tightness of the gastric band.

Minor surgical complications, including wound infections and risks for minor bleeding, only occur in 10% of patients. (WebMD, n.d.)

As opposed to gastric bypass surgery, gastric banding doesn't prevent your body from absorbing food whatsoever, which means that you won't have to worry about experiencing any vitamin or mineral loss in your body.

Types of Gastric Banding Techniques Used in Hypnotherapy for Weight Loss

• Sleeve Gastrectomy - This procedure involves physically removing half of a patient's stomach to leave behind space, which is usually the size of a banana. When this part of the stomach is taken out, it cannot be reversed. This may seem like one of the most extreme types of gastric band surgeries, and due to its level of extremity, it also presents a lot of risks. When the reasons why the sleeve Gastrectomy is done and gets reviewed, it may not seem worth it. However, it has become one of the most popular methods used in surgery, as a restrictive means of reducing a patient's appetite. It is particularly helpful to those who suffer from obesity. It has a high success rate with very few complications, according to medical practitioners. Those who have had the surgery have experienced losing up to 50% of their total weight, which is quite a lot for someone suffering from obesity. It is equally helpful to those who suffer from compulsive eating disorders, like binge eating. When you have the procedure done, your surgeon will make either a very large or a few small incisions in the abdomen. The physical recovery of this procedure may take up to six weeks. (WebMD, n.d.)

• Vertical banded Gastroplasty - This gastric band procedure, also known as VBG, involves the same band used during the sleeve Gastrectomy, which is placed around the stomach. The stomach is then stapled above the band to form a small pouch, which in some sense shrinks the stomach to produce the same effects. The procedure has been noted as a successful one to lose weight compared to many other types of weight-loss surgeries. Even though compared to the Sleeve Gastrectomy, it may seem like a less complicated surgery, it has a higher complication rate. That is why it is considered far less common. Until today, there are only 5% of bariatric surgeons perform this particular gastric band surgery. Nevertheless, it is known for producing results and can still be used in hypnotherapy to produce similar results without the complications.

• Mixed Surgery (Restrictive and Malabsorptive) - This type of gastric band surgery forms a crucial part of most types of weight-loss surgeries. It is more commonly referred to as gastric bypass and is done first, prior to other weight-loss surgeries. It also involves stapling the stomach and creates a shape of an intestine down the line of your stomach. This is done to ensure the patient consumes less food, referred to as restrictive mixed surgery, combined with Malabsorptive surgery, meaning to absorb less food in the body.

What You Need to Know About Hypnotic Gastric Band Therapy

If you're wondering whether gastric band surgery is right for you, you may want to consider getting the hypnotherapy version thereof. Hypnotherapy is the perfect alternative, it is 100% safe as opposed to surgery, which has many complications, and also a lot more affordable. It has a success rate of more than 90% in patients, which is why more people prefer it over gastric band surgery. Given that you can also conduct it in the comfort of your own home, you don't even have to worry about the cost involved. Overall it serves as a very convenient way to slim down, essentially shrinking your stomach.

Again, hypnosis doesn't involve any physical procedure involving surgery. It is a safe alternative that uses innovative and developed technology to help you get where you want to be. The hypnotherapy session involves visualizing a virtual gastric band being fitted around your stomach that allows you to have the same experience as you initially would during surgery, but without the discomfort, excessive costs, and inconvenience.

The effect is feeling as if you are hungry for longer periods, require less food, and experiencing a feeling of being full, even if you've only eaten half of your regular-sized portion. This will also help you make healthier choices and discover that you can indeed develop a much healthier relationship with food than you currently have.

If you're wondering whether gastric band hypnotherapy will work for you, you have to ask yourself whether you have the imagination to support your session. Now, of course, everybody has an imagination, but is yours reasonable enough?

If you can close your eyes and imagine yourself looking at something in front of you that is not there, and spend time focusing on it, then you can make it through gastric band hypnotherapy successfully.

It's normal to think before you start anything that if it isn't tailored to you specifically, it is likely to fail. However, visual gastric band hypnosis can offer you emotional healing. This supports your goals, including weight loss and health restoration. If you spend time engaging in it, you will learn that you can achieve whatever you set your intention on. You can remove your cravings subconsciously, eliminate any negative and emotional stress, as well as memories that form a part of your emotional eating pattern. Given that emotionality forms a big part of weight gain, you should know that it can be removed from your conscious mind through hypnotherapy and serve any individual willing to try it.

Gastric band hypnotherapy has a 95% success rate among patients, according to a clinical study conducted in the U.K. This study also proved that most people will be able to accept and succeed in hypnotherapy, but if they're not open to the experience, they won't find it helpful at all. People who are too closed off from new ideas, like hypnotherapy, which is often made out to be a negative practice among the uneducated, won't be able to relax properly for a hypnotherapist's words to take effect. (Engle, 2019)

After just one hypnotherapy session, you will know if it works, as it is supposed to start working after just one session. That is why hypnotherapy is not recommended for everyone. It's only suggested to anyone ready to change their feelings toward food. If you don't believe in it or that it will get you to where you want to go on your weight loss journey, it is deemed useless.

The cost of gastric band hypnotherapy sessions with a professional hypnotherapist can only be established after you've undergone an evaluation. Usually, every new patient requires up to five sessions in person. During these sessions, energy therapy techniques are also taught, which will help assist any struggle a patient may have with anxiety, anger, stress, and any other negative emotion.

CHAPTER 12:

Mind and Body Connection

People who experience disease, accidents and other trauma to their bodies often react by dissociating themselves from painful sensations and physical self-awareness. While this can be beneficial in the short term, it can also conflict with a person's ability to self-regulate and create meaningful behavioral improvements.

Obesity is a source of depression in itself, and weight loss consumers still detach from their bodies-this This is one explanation that they can over-eat and not be aware of actual satiation signals. When it comes to patterns and behaviors that may not benefit the development of well-being in general, parts of the body may respond negatively, given the individual's conscious intention to do otherwise.

Our mission is not only to teach customers about their mind-body connectivity, which happens to be bi-directional but to help them become more adept at using it as a healing tool. Because of this two-way function, we can take a "top-down" approach, change a person's way of thinking and feeling to affect changes in their physiology, or take a "bottom-up" tact physical functions to improve the thoughts and emotional state of a person.

Another approach I help clients work towards enhancing their awareness and responding to their bodies' signals and building self-acceptance is to use a massage on the abdomen. This strategy will also help overcome stomach issues that encourage unhealthy eating and drinking, or even traumatic conditions.

The abdomen is genuinely an energy source, a powerhouse in itself. The Japanese call this center of our body "hara," a place where "ki," or energy, is produced. During my martial arts training, I learned to embrace and focus on this part of my body, and once I did, I broke through some previous mental and physical limitations.

Releasing unhelpful discomfort in the abdomen can relax the entire body and mind, with several positive outcomes resulting:

1) Reduces chronic stress and anxiety and alleviates pain

2) Increases metabolism and enhances intestinal fires

3) Builds self-acceptance

4) Strengthens the connection between mind and body and increases awareness of physical sensations

Meditation for Mindful Hypnosis of the Heart

For individual communities like ours, people are admonished to "suck for your belly at a young age! "(Do you unintentionally keep stress in yours right now?!) Regardless of height and weight, we are full of self-awareness in this part of the body and feel inside. As a result, we are often detached from our heart and may have pessimistic feelings about it.

Even if a person doesn't struggle to be overweight, they can "keep" the gut unconsciously in a strengthened, restricted role. Practicing this belly exercise will make the enteric nervous system-the digestive tract-transition towards a "remembered health" more relaxed.

Sit quiet, with your eyes closed. Take your thoughts to the middle area, to your heart. Let yourself aware of how you feel about that part of your body. Let the emotions, concepts, and opinions rise into your consciousness, like bubbles flowing from the sea. Do not be your feelings; just watch them unfold. You can experience hearing your voice or hearing specific thoughts in someone else's voice as well. Just watch them as they float up.

You should count your breath as you breathe in, count as you catch your breath, and count as you breathe out. Using the diaphragm, you want to live heavily, and your abdomen inflates more than your chest region. It is a simple way to help the conscious mind shift away from disturbing or disruptive thoughts and activate relaxation. You might want to apply some imagery to it, including seeing a number written in sand and seeing a gentle wave wash it away, replacing it with the next number. And you can want to consider the numbers in your head.

Note when you do so that the stomach muscles are relaxed and other body muscles relax as they do. Just when your stomach settles, does it become possible to dissipate the pain in your body fades away? A surge of warmth passes over you and helps your mind to become calm, peaceful.

Then raise your right hand to the top of your uterus, gently resting it just below your bra line. Pressing gently in a clockwise direction, start rotating it to the left. It should rub your belly's outer circumference gently, reaching up to the tops of the arms, falling to the bottom of the navel, and then reversing the other hand. Your skin and flesh move by gentle pressure but will not feel uncomfortable.

Imagine that as you massage your "hara," you activate and balance the life-force within you. You link inside this personal, intense center. When you find that there are troubling thoughts or emotions, let them float both up and down. Consider that something that blocks, inhibits, or otherwise harms you is being dislodged and discharged.

Begin to breathe deeply and rhythmically, inhale excellent, soothing substances, and exhale all that isn't beneficial or curative. Imagine your healthy, fully working digestive tract, returned to optimal fitness. Bring in a state of peace, a state of well-being, just though you experience revitalization and regeneration of the energies within your heart.

When you've done 10-12 massage rotations, relax and indulge in the sensations of relaxation and calm now, realizing that you'll experience the good benefits of having this unique period as you return to your usual activities.

Spend a few minutes a day in abdominal yoga, and you will realize after a short time that not only the abdomen and overall body will feel better, but the digestive system will also change!

Body Parts

We may also use a method called "Body Parts" to enhance the connection between mind and body. This approach can be a stand-alone strategy, or it can quickly improve specific techniques you use to assist a customer. Ultimately, it acts as an excellent method to attract and expand a customer for future research. It helps to build hope that you will "open the door" between a person's aware and subconscious minds, encouraging them to connect openly to aspects of themselves that will be part of a "unit" of recovery.

Start with inducing some consumer concentration and relaxation. You can make them concentrate on breathing; they can place their attention on a hand or leg, leading them to close their eyes and finding they can still imagine that portion of their body, even with their eyes closed. The key goal is to focus their attention on their physical self.

Using something similar from here, like:

When you learn your side, now you may think about all the stuff the side does with you how it supports you in so many ways: touching, stroking, squeezing, grabbing, raising, folding, feeding (describing every client-relevant tasks)

A beautiful hand is a hand. I wonder if you should say what you think of what it does for you?

PAUSE

So, if the hand were able to talk, what would it tell you? And what is it you need?

PAUSE

That's right, and talk of your heart now, please the incredible pump the allows blood to circulate to keep you healthy. Your wonderful heart built to beat so many times in your lifetime. Nobody knows exactly how many cycles it is, but it works to achieve the beats for you. Who do you want your heart to tell?

PAUSE

So, what does the heart want to tell you about what it's going through about what you need? Hear it now.

PAUSE

That's right, and now just talk of your big toe on your left foot (* or some other, untouched part of your body, maybe an eyebrow or an ear)

That's helping you keep calm to make you walk. Your beautiful big toe builds to help you make more strides in your life.

No one knows precisely how many steps this is, but it works to do the number of moves for you. I'm curious if you will let yourself be overwhelmed with admiration of how good the toe works for you and will continue to.

PAUSE

So, would the toe like to talk to (any part of the body which needs healing) now? Should this happen, what will they tell each other?

PAUSE

Could you imagine pretend if you have to that all the well-being in that toe transmit in any way maybe even the code for that well-being can be replicated and pasted anywhere throughout the body it's needed now (provide patter explaining where and how it's required?

That's right, so now think about your lungs, those magnificent lungs that draw in and filter fresh oxygen for you to keep you healthy. The excellent lungs build to breathe in and out too many times in the lifetime. Well, no one knows just how many times it is, but they are trying to satisfy the number of breaths for you.

PAUSE

So, what do the lungs want to tell you what they're going through what they need from you?

I might recommend that a client needs a real chat about their knees and liver in any area of the body that has suffered through lifestyle decisions. I may even encourage the client to get support with their hands, who are often involved in poor eating habits, to function more closely towards their objectives.

Following these conversations, suggest that ALL parts of the body integrate, as part of the whole ... working together towards wellness, promoting comfort, balance, healing, continued enlightenment and improvement, etc.

* With a few tactics, we will put in a balanced body part:

1. In a diversion to the cycle from dealing with the negative side of being overweight or obese, it momentarily focuses away from what is wrong with the body.

2. As a resource for body parts that need healing.

Every part of the body is negatively affected by the extra weight and should approach it this way. Having room for an interactive conversation with a person and their body will provide them with knowledge, perspective, and inspiration and promote calming reactions within the body.

CHAPTER 13:

Gastric Band Hypnosis Training

The physical gastric band requires a surgical procedure that involves reducing the size of your stomach pocket to accommodate less volume of food and, as a result of the stretching of the walls of the stomach, send signals to the brain that you are filled and therefore need to stop eating any further.

The hypnotic gastric band also works in the same manner, although in this case the only surgical tools you will need are your mind and your body, and the great part is you can conduct the procedure yourself.

The hypnotic gastric band also conditions your mind and body to restrict excess consumption of food after very modest meals.

There are three specific differences between the surgical (physical) and hypnotic gastric bands:

- In using the hypnotic band, all necessary adjustments are made by continued use of trance.

- There is an absence of physical surgery and therefore you are exposed to no risks at all.

- When compared with the surgical gastric band, the hypnotic gastric band is a lot cheaper and easier to do.

How Hypnosis Improves Communication between Stomach and Brain

How would you know when you have had enough to eat? Initially, you will begin to feel the weight and area of the food. When your stomach is full, the food presses against and extends the stomach well, and the nerve endings in the walls of the stomach respond. When these nerves are stimulated, they transfer a signal to the brain, and we get the feeling of satiety.

And, as the stomach fills up and food enters the digestive tract, PYY and GLP-1 is released and trigger a feeling of satiety in the brain that additionally prompts us to quit eating.

Sadly, when individuals always overeat, they become desensitized to both the nerve signals and the neuropeptide signaling system. During the initial installation trance, we use hypnotic and images to re-sensitize the brain to these signs. Your hypnotic band restores the full effect of these nervous and neuropeptide messages. With the benefits of hypnotic in view, we can recalibrate this system and increase your sensitivity to these signs, so you feel full and truly satisfied when you have eaten enough to fill that little pouch at the top of your stomach.

A hypnotic gastric band causes your body to carry on precisely as if you have carried out a surgical operation. It contracts your stomach and adjusts the signals from your stomach to your brain, so you feel full rapidly. The hypnotic band uses a few uncommon attributes of hypnotic. As a matter of first importance, hypnotic permits us to talk to parts of the body and mind that are not under conscious control. Interestingly as it might appear, in a trance, we can really convince the body to carry on distinctively even though our conscious mind has no methods for coordinating that change.

The Power of the Gastric Band

A renowned and dramatic case of the power of hypnotic to influence our bodies directly is in the emergency treatment of burns. A few doctors have used hypnotic on many occasions to accelerate and improve the recuperating of extreme injuries and to help reduce the excruciating pains for their patients. If somebody is seriously burnt, there will be damage to the tissue, and the body reacts with inflammation. The patients are hypnotized to forestall the soreness. His patients heal quite rapidly and with less scarring.

There are a lot more instances of how the mind can directly and physically influence the body. We realize that chronic stress can cause stomach ulcers, and a psychological shock can turn somebody's hair to grey color overnight. In any case, what I especially like about this aspect of hypnotism is that it is an archived case of how the mind influences the body positively and medically. It will be somewhat of a miraculous event if the body can get into a hypnotic state that can cause significant physical changes in your body. Hypnotic trance without anyone else has a profound physiological effect. The most immediate effect is that subjects discover it deeply relaxing. Interestingly, the most widely recognized perception that my customers report after I have seen them—regardless of what we have been dealing with—is that their loved ones tell them they look more youthful.

Cybernetic Loop

Your brain and body are in constant correspondence in a cybernetic loop: they continually influence one another. As the mind unwinds in a trance, so too does the body. When the body unwinds, it feels good, and it sends that message to the brain, which thus feels healthier and unwinds much more. This procedure decreases stress and makes more energy accessible to the immune system of the body. It is essential to take note that the remedial effects of hypnotic don't require tricks or amnesia. For example, burns patients realize they have been burnt, so they don't need to deny the glaring evidence of how burnt parts of their bodies are. He essentially hypnotizes them and requests that they envision cool, comfortable sensations over the burnt area. That imaginative activity changes their body's response to the burns.

The enzymes that cause inflammation are not released, and accordingly, the burn doesn't advance to a more elevated level of damage, and there is reduced pain during the healing process.

By using hypnotic and imagery, a doctor can get his patients' bodies to do things that are totally outside their conscious control. Willpower won't make these sorts of changes, but the creative mind is more grounded than the will. By using hypnotic and imagery to talk to the conscious mind, we can have a physiological effect in as little as 20 minutes. In my work, I recently had another phenomenal idea of how hypnotic can accelerate the body's normal healing process. I worked with a soldier in the Special Forces who experienced extreme episodes of skin inflammation (eczema). He revealed to me that the quickest recuperation he had ever made from an eczema episode was six days. I realized that the way toward healing is a natural sequence of events carried out by various systems within the body, so I hypnotized him and, while in a trance, requested that his conscious mind follow precisely the same process that it regularly uses to heal his eczema, however, to do everything quicker.

One and a half days after, the eczema was gone. With hypnotic, we can enormously enhance the effect of the mind. When we fit your hypnotic gastric band, we are using the very same strategy of hypnotic correspondence to the conscious mind. We communicate to the brain with distinctive imagery, and the brain alters your body's responses, changing your physical response to food so your stomach is constricted, and you feel truly full after only a few.

What Makes the Hypnotic Work So Well?

A few people think that it's difficult to accept that trance and imagery can have such an extreme and ground-breaking effect. Some doctors were at first distrustful and accepted that his patients more likely than not had fewer burns than was written in their medical records, because the cures he effected had all the earmarks of being close to marvelous. It took quite a long while, and numerous exceptional remedies before such work were generally understood and acknowledged.

Once in a while, the cynic and the patient are the same individuals. We need the results, but we battle to accept that it truly will work. At the conscious level, our minds are very much aware of the contrast between what we imagine and physical reality. In any case, another astounding hypnotic marvel shows that it doesn't make a difference what we accept at the conscious level since trance permits our mind to react to a reality that is independent of what we deliberately think. This phenomenon is classified as "trance logic."

Trance logic was first recognized 50 years ago by a renowned researcher of hypnotic named Dr. Martin Orne, who worked for a long time at the University of Pennsylvania. Dr. Orne directed various tests that demonstrated that in hypnotic, individuals could carry on as though two absolutely opposing facts were valid simultaneously. In one study, he hypnotized a few people so they couldn't see a seat he put directly before them. Then he requested that they walk straight ahead. The subjects all swerved around the seat.

Notwithstanding, when examined regarding the chair, they reported there was nothing there. They couldn't see the seat. Some of them even denied that they had swerved by any means. They accepted they were telling the truth when they said they couldn't see the seat, but at another level, their bodies realized it was there and moved to abstain from hitting it.

The test showed that hypnotic permits the mind to work at the same time on two separate levels, accepting two isolated, opposing things. It is possible to be hypnotized and have a hypnotic gastric band fitted but then to "know" with your conscious mind that you don't have surgical scars and you don't have a physical gastric band embedded. Trance logic implies that a part of your mind can trust one thing, and another part can accept the direct opposite, and your mind and body can continue working, accepting that two unique things are valid. So, you will be capable to consciously realize that you have not paid a huge amount of dollars for a surgical process, but then at the deepest level of unconscious command, your body accepts that you have a gastric band and will act in like manner. Subsequently, your stomach is conditioned to signal "feeling full" to your brain after only a couple of mouthfuls. So, you feel satisfied, and you get to lose more weight.

Visualization Is Easier Than You Think

The hypnotic we use to make your gastric band uses "visualization" and "influence loaded imager." Visualization is the creation of pictures in your mind. We would all be able to do it. It is an interesting part of the reasoning. For instance, think about your front door and ask yourself which side the lock is on. To address that question, you see an image in your mind's eye. It doesn't make a difference at all how reasonable or bright the image is, it is only how your mind works, and you see as much as you have to see. Influence loaded imagery is the psychological term for genuinely significant pictures. In this process, we use pictures in the mind's eye that have emotional significance.

Although hypnotic recommendations are incredible, they are dramatically upgraded by ground-breaking images when we are communicating directly to the body. For instance, you will be unable to accelerate your heart just by telling it to beat faster. Still, if you envision remaining on a railroad line and seeing a train surging towards you, your heart accelerates pretty quickly. Your body overreacts to clear, meaningful pictures.

CHAPTER 14:

Weight Management Program

Well, there are some other effective ways in which an individual can lose weight. You might decide to combine them to make the processes faster and more manageable. What meditation does is that it will help you enhance some of these factors. You may find that the activities you chose to undertake become more effective as you conduct them. We do not disregard the methods; we only recommend that you complement them with meditation.

In some cases, you find that mediation can be useful on its own. While in other cases, you have to combine it with other activities to help an individual struggling with weight loss. We will go through some of the other things that you might need to look at as you get on a weight loss journey. Below are some of them.

Dieting

This is perhaps the first thing we think of any time we think of weight loss. We gain weight as a result of the poor eating habits that we adapt, and they cost us a lot. Eating wrong does not only make us add weight, but it can also affect our health.

We have some diseases that result from eating unhealthy foods. Plant-based meals tend to be nutritious and, at times, provide the best solution for weight loss. We shall discuss three weight-loss diets that an individual can utilize to lose weight.

Ketogenic Diet

A keto diet is a low carb diet. It utilizes the concept of consuming high fat and the required amount of proteins while also taking a low carb diet. Carbohydrates are mainly composed of sugars. When we increase their consumption, we have excess sugars in the bloodstream that cannot be converted into energy. In the process, your body converts it into fats, and you end up gaining weight. A keto diet helps an individual lose weight by lowering the intake of carbohydrates. You only consume what your body requires; hence, no sugar needs to be converted into fats. You find that while using this diet, you can also burn the excess fats in your body. This works in a process known as ketosis. When the intake of glucose and other sugars is low, the body begins to convert the fats in the body into energy. When this process occurs consistently, you can manage to get rid of all the excess fats, and as a result, you lose weight.

Paleo Diet

Its name was generated from the fact that it was the diet used during the Paleolithic era. If you have studied history, you probably know the events that occurred in this particular period. During such times, there were no processed foods, and people would eat vegetables, fruits, seeds, nuts, and meat. In that era, there was barely any obesity case since people ate what they planted or what they hunted. People came up with the ideology that if that type of diet helped people keep fit, then it can be an excellent diet to adapt to this era. Much of the weight gain is as a result of consuming food substances that are processed. They have no nutritious benefits to our bodies; instead, we drink a lot of food that has no use. We get full and satisfied after the meal, yet the body does not utilize the food. We end up gaining extra weight with no nutritious benefit. With the help of a Paleo diet, you get to consume that which you need. The body utilizes the food consumed to the maximum, and in the end, you keep fit and barely add extra weight.

Mediterranean Diet

The main inspiration behind a Mediterranean diet comes from the eating habits of the people living in the Mediterranean region. Some of the countries involved were Italy and Greece. Their menu was composed of fruits, unrefined cereals, vegetables, olive oil, and legumes. It also included some moderate consumption of meat, animal by-products, and wine. People using this diet were found to be healthy due to the nutrients contained in the food that they consumed. It was challenging to get diseases that result from poor eating habits. Lifestyle diseases were difficult to come by, especially this type of diet. The diet helps an individual lose weight since they get to take up what is required by the body. It also ensures that they maintain their weight. While taking this diet, you lower your carbohydrate intake. This means that you reduce the sugar levels in your bloodstream and that what you eat is what you require. Your body acquires the right amount of sugars, so there are no excess sugars that need to be converted into fats. That is how the Mediterranean diet helps you lose weight and have a healthy body.

How Does Meditation Help While Dieting?

You might be wondering how meditation can help while dieting and ensuring that you lose weight. Dieting can be difficult, especially if you are not disciplined enough to do so. You might find yourself having some regular cheat days, which may appear more recurrently than they should. You find that you are regularly doing this and end up not dieting at all. Meditation brings you into realizing some of the poor decisions that you make as far as eating is concerned. As a result, you can make better decisions once you understand where you went wrong. Dieting can be challenging, and you need to stay focused for you to manage to complete the diet successfully.

If you are dieting to lose weight, you need to observe the food every single day keenly. This is to help you ensure that the dieting will be useful in accomplishing its purpose. In the beginning, you will face a lot of temptations, but you can manage them with the aid of meditation. It ensures that you stay focused on the goal, and you manage to lose weight as planned.

Exercise

You might be the type of individual that immediately thinks of the gym anytime you hear about losing weight. You could believe that there is something that you physically need to do to cut off the weight. In the process, you might acquire a gym membership, and you set a gym routine whereby you get to go to the gym at certain times during the day. Even while exercising, you need meditation. Meditation allows you to concentrate on the various activities that you are undertaking. In the process, you get to give your full energy into the activities that you are taking. You find that even the various exercises that you engage in become useful in helping you lose weight. It allows you to burn the extra fats and maintains a good shape.

There is a lot of incredible power in meditation. In that calm state of mind, incredible things happen. It more like a magical occurrence. Your account becomes keen and focused on the things that matter. In the process, you find that your performance levels are increased as you make better decisions regarding the issues at hand. This may seem like an easy thing to do, but we barely do it. An individual may find the process of meditation tedious for them to handle, yet it requires a small amount of your time. At that moment, you get to relax your mind as you think of the conditions around you. During your gym time, as you are busy exercising, you can use some of that time to meditate. This will improve your concentration and can, at times, cause you to be energized. The process of exercising can get tiring, and you need to find a way to ease the burden that comes with it. With meditation, this is easily achievable.

Consuming the Necessary Amount of Food

At the time, we waste a lot of food that is not necessary. You only find that you eat because there is food to be consumed and not because you need it. With the help of meditation, there is a lot that you can accomplish. Eating when there is no need to can lead to weight gain. Your body keeps taking foods in excess quantities that it does not need. As this process progresses, you find yourself adding a lot of weight. Meditation will help you avoid some of these incidences by helping you make the right decisions. When it comes to eating, you only do so when it is necessary.

You can plan your meals and the amount you wish to consume at a given time in a day. For instance, during breakfast, you might decide to eat a heavy meal. This is to provide you with the strength that you need to tackle the day. Breakfast is an essential meal, so you are allowed to eat slightly more than the other meals. During lunchtime, you can eat a slightly smaller portion than that of breakfast.

On the other hand, at night, you can ensure that you take the smallest part. At night there is no significant activity to be carried out unless you are working a night shift. The recommended amount you should consume should be just enough to carry you through the night. In between the day, you can include some small snacks and ensure that they are healthy snacks. If you manage to follow this keenly, your weight loss journey will be effortless. Meditation will play a significant role in ensuring that you consume the amount of food that is necessary and according to your meal plan.

Healthy Eating Habits

There are certain habits that we adapt to, and that contributes to weight gain. For instance, you might have a habit of eating too fast, and as a result, food is not well processed. This causes the food to become waste, and instead of benefiting your body, it becomes a problem for your organization. In some situations, you might find that what you consumed had some nutritious benefits, but due to your poor eating habits, it does not help you in the way that it should. At times, you might cook a lot of food or even serve yourself a lot of food. You might get to a point whereby you feel like you are already full. However, you keep eating because there is food on your plate or because you have some leftover food. The excess food you consume once you are full will not help your body, so you can find yourself adding weight.

CHAPTER 15:

Gastric Band Techniques

Placing

In this meditation, you will learn how to walk along a beautiful beach walk, allowing you and deeply relax.

Follow me on this mental vacation as we place an emotional and mental, and gastric band around your stomach, which will allow you to feel full as soon as you eat exactly as much food as you need.

So, get into a comfortable seated position, on your favorite spot, so that you are undisturbed for the rest of this session. As you relax, the gastric band will become more powerful and influential over your life. Take a big deep breath, relax, and then exhale the tension and worry as you close your eyes. Feel your body already slowing down. Take another breath and let to go with a sigh of relief. This moment is for you to practice your new lifestyle, of being full, at the perfect time. Now say to you with faith, "overeating is impossible for me."

Now breathe into the truth of these words as you breathe them out into reality. You are creating a smaller stomach. Relax and breathe, and then use the power of your imagination to visualize a beautiful beach with white sand, reflecting in the sunlight. It looks like snow. You can see the turquoise waters fading to a deep blue as the ocean goes deeper.

Look down into the sand where you stand, and notice the beautiful bits of shells with all different colors and textures as you see dried seaweed scattered about something that catches your eye buried into the sand, it is your preferred color. So, as you get closer, you will see that it is a small yet thick band that is as big around as your fist, and it just so happens that it is the most vivid version of your favorite color. The brightness of this hue brings you joy. The curious, round band, flashing of your most beloved color choice is called the gastric band

It is placed around the top of your stomach, cinching down the amount your stomach can hold. So, it makes your stomach feel smaller, which gives you that feeling of fullness that you've had enough to eat. This band only exists in the medical world. But you can get the same results, using the power of your mind, by placing the band within and around your stomach in this relaxing session.

Feel your feet entering the sand and allow yourself on each step to relax more and more. Notice the powdery texture, dispersing under your feet, and allow it deeply soothe you. Feel the ocean breeze, and smell the salty air. As you walk, you will get tired. A perfect chair has appeared just for you, facing the ocean. So have a seat and recline backward with your gastric band in your hand. Familiarize yourself with its shape and size. It is like a small belt that can be tightened and loosened.

This relaxing gastric band session brings you to perfect health and weight through the power of your mind. It brings about a new and improved positive attitude to life with intention, positivity, and knowing when enough is enough. Now bring your hands into the mode of prayer and notice how you feel. Notice your mind and body going back on track, firmly ready to eat the healthy amount.

Take a few calming, relaxing moments before coming back to the present moment. Take a long breath in and feel the gastric band as it's limiting your ability to overeat. Feel the band affecting the weight throughout your body. When you are ready, just gently open your eyes. And then seal this in with a grateful smile.

Tightening

Welcome to this relaxing meditation. This meditation will guide you to a pristine lake that is surrounded by mountains and help you to tighten your gastric band, making for an even smaller stomach that will fill up quickly. Get yourself into a nice seated position where you can easily fully let go, and you will not be disturbed by the surrounding world.

As you get into a powerful state of relaxation, begin to imagine that you are tightening this gastric band, and as you do so, you will find that weight-loss becomes easier and easier by the day. Now begin to breathe deeply while allowing your body to expand. Exhale all of your stress out and take another deep breath in, and as you exhale and allow, let your eyes gently closed.

Now notice how you feel. Notice how your body is settling down and as it becomes relaxed as we go along. Let go of any current worries or obligations. Enjoying for yourself, and you begin your health and wellness journey from the first session by placing a gastric band near your stomach with the power of your mind. So, appreciate yourself for taking on this amazing opportunity.

Now say to yourself, "I will eat only as much food as I need. I need less food to feel full."

Breath in, and allow these words to become part of every level of your awareness. Breathe out any doubt and breathe in any truth that you are capable of eating just the right amount to have the perfect shape, size, and overall wellness. Now relax, calm down, and be at complete ease. Let your body slow down just a little bit more. Activate your imagination by bringing into your mind the eye, the site of a magnificent lake that is surrounded by mountains. And the sky, which is a crisp turquoise blue dappled with the cloud. And the sun is shining all around you. The waters of this lake are crystal clear, and it's reflecting the blueness of the sky. The water is acting as a mirror for the mountain range.

Now become aware of your stomach and notice it becoming smaller from your wonderful session on the beach when you first found your gastric band. Feel how your stomach is comfortable and happy about its new size and wants to become even smaller.

As you walk toward the lake, notice the soil under your feet, becoming smooth and supportive. As you go near to the water edge, dip your toes in the cool and fresh aqua. Even though your feet are submerged, the waters of this mystical lake relax your entire body.

Notice beside you the small red canoe waiting for you. Enter into this canoe and pick up the beautiful hand-carved oar. The oar signifies the ability to be able to tighten your gastric band. Dip the oar into the water, moving to the bottom of the lake, and push off the shore. Feel as this simple movement helps to tighten your gastric band by a millimeter.

Also, visualize yourself in your kitchen now preparing your next meal. You will find that when you put the plate on your food, all of your choices are healthy. You will notice that you will only scoop a small amount of each item because you have a good ability to put the right amount of food that you need on your plate, now with your gastric band supporting you. You don't want to waste a bite of food. You should only eat the perfect amount.

See yourself eating this healthy meal and shocked at the small food that it took for you to feel satisfied. Now, as you rise from this wonderful meditation, allow the image of the canoe and the see-through water to fade away from your mind, as well as the great mountains and along with the visual of your next meal.

Right now, bring yourself back from this experience into reality. Breathe in deeply, and become aware of your surroundings in the present moment. Wiggle around your toes and fingers a little bit and feel the fresh new energy and wisdom coming into you. And then, whenever you are ready, open your eyes.

Removal

So far, you have placed this band around your stomach while walking on the relaxing beach and tightening the band while rowing your canoe on a crystal-clear lake. Right now, we will visit an ancient Japanese castle to be able to remove this band and discard it during the beautiful ceremony. Now make sure that you're in a comfortable position, in a place that you can enjoy practicing this relaxing session. This is the final step in your gastric band experience. So, take a nice deep breath in and then breathe out while closing your eyes.

Relax your body. Feel it sinking into the chair or bed, soft and supportive underneath you.

Breathe in and then breathe out while noticing the gentle rise and fall of your chest as you breathe in. Now start becoming aware of your abdomen and feel how slim it is as you're, eating less food. You are becoming fuller and making hunger outdated. You know that you're supposed to eat, but eating doesn't consume your day or your mind. You only eat when you should eat and refuse to eat when you don't should eat. It's as simple as that.

Activate your creative mind again. Now imagine that you are standing in a beautiful field with tall grass, blowing in your wind. Now imagine that there's a path in front of you, and that path is made up of smooth stones. As you walk along this path, see yourself coming towards a magnificent Japanese temple that was built hundreds of years ago.

The building is well maintained with a fresh coat made of red paint as well as gold trim surrounding the windows and doors. Now make your way up to the front door and feel like the iron handle in your hand on this door is massive as you open it.

So, as you step inside the temple, feel the cool air around you. Also, imagine that the interior of this structure is a work of art, crafted by sheer genius. Now notice that there is a large golden bowl in the center of the room that is set atop a marble column. Now, as you move away from this bowl, it will appear to be illuminated with a ray of sunlight, which is casting down through the window on the rooftop.

As you see, the, reflecting the light like a diamond. Now, you easily remove the gastric band and place it inside the sacred water. So, you can see that it is your favorite color, yet it's a bit worn and tired from all the work that it did for your health. Now imagine the ray of light beaming down and see it begin to dissolve the gastric band until the water is pure. Start to feel lighter than ever, and your stomach smaller, along with your figure, shrinking every day.

Feel the sensations of touch at your fingertips. Move your focus to your abdomen and to all your vital organs. Notice how your belly feels and how it is digesting. Notice your pelvis and hips and the sensations of your weight as it's pressing it down. This should take you into a deeper state of relaxation. Your awareness should go down on each leg, over your knees, move down all the way to your feet, and touch each toe.

CHAPTER 16:

Virtual Gastric Band Sample

Start breathing slowly and deeply.

-

you are lying down, and you are entirely receptive to me

-

You hear my voice mix with your inner voice.

-

My voice is now your voice.

-

Breathe in through your nose and out through your mouth.

Let it create circular and continuous breathing.

-

Feel the air flowing in, filling the lower lungs.

The abdomen swells to the maximum inhalation, so hold your breath for three seconds. Then mentally count to five when you exhale.

-

Follow me:

Inhale deeply 1,2,3.

Exhale slowly: 1, 2, 3, 4, 5.

-

Inhale 1,2,3.

exhale: 1, 2, 3, 4, 5.

-

Every time you exhale, you feel more and more relaxed.

-

Inhale 1,2,3.

exhale: 1, 2, 3, 4, 5.

-

Every time you exhale, you feel more and more relaxed.

-

It will help you think much more clearly by increasing the level of oxygen reaching your brain.

-

you are perfectly calm and relaxed

-

As you continue to breathe and relax, you know your feet and calves' muscles are becoming heavy and comfortable. Let go of the tension and stiffness.

And this pleasant feeling of relaxation begins to spread to your leg muscles. You can go deeper and deeper.

-

I am feeling peaceful and calm.

-

You are perfectly calm and relaxed.

-

You can go deeper and deeper.

-

Feel the sensation in your feet

-

feel the force of gravity pushing them down.

let them go.

-

They are heavily relaxed.

-

Your calves are also massive.

The force of gravity brings them down.

And you also begin to feel heavy and motionless legs.

Perfectly relaxed

you are calm and relaxed.

.

This feeling of relaxation diffuses in the body

-

And every muscle in the abdomen and chest becomes calm and relaxed, free from tension and rigidity.

-

This sensation spreads to the muscles of the back, and the muscles become relaxed and relaxed.

-

Along the spine, the muscles become relaxed and relaxed. One by one. Like a mental massage from the base of the spine to the neck.

-

With every word I say, you feel more relaxed.

-

Go deeper and deeper

-

Enjoy this unique moment where you get inside yourself and get stronger and stronger.

-

This feeling of relaxation spreads to the shoulders and arms.

your right arm is heavy

-

Now your left arm is also massive.

-

Let go of any stiffness, and you may notice a tingling sensation on your fingertips as your arms relax.

-

You feel heavy and relaxed

-

You keep going deeper and deeper

-

Now let go of your thoughts and feel your neck muscles relax entirely, all the way to your head.

-

You're calm and safe, at peace with yourself.

And the tension in your forehead simply begins to melt away.

-

The muscles of the eyebrows are relaxed and relaxed

-

More and more deeply

In a few moments, I'll count from 1 to 3.

When I get to 3, your mind will be ten times calmer and more relaxed

-

Let's start: 1...2...3...

-

A positive feeling spread in you

-

Today will be a special day for you.

The day of the intervention has finally arrived.

-

You find yourself lying on a trolley in a

white surgery room

-

you know you are going to

be changed and that when you wake up you

will be different

-

you will be starting a new life

-

you see figures in green around

you

-

They are slowly moving

-

they are relaxed and perfectly know what they are doing.

Today they will help you change your life.

They are talking to you, asking you to relax, and gently placing a mask on your face

-

you almost feel a hand on your wrist briefly

and you're vaguely aware of the

noises around you and the ceiling lights

-

you're happy at this moment and

somehow you sense something happening on

your tummy

-

you feel something gently spread across

your skin

A slight sensation of pressure and you

can sense that

something is happening inside you.

-

You are inside you and see a white rubber band tie around your stomach, which is now as small as a golf ball.

-

it has all plan with the

greatest of care you feel it is

tested and checked

-

and there's a feeling

of satisfaction in the air

-

it's all over

-

the band fits now, and you can visualize

that band pinched around the entrance

of the stomach

-

That band means a lot to you.

-

You feel safe and secure now.

-

You already feel a sense of contentment and satiety.

-

your new life has just begun

-

You are in front of the mirror.

-

You can see and feel that something is profoundly different.

-

you can feel something different in

your stomach,

there's a tightness there

-

Remember how you used to feel

when did you know you had overeating?

-

remember how it used to have that feel,

and from now on, the smallest bit of food

feels huge

-

your stomach feels full all the time

-

Your life is so good because you've lost weight, and you start to notice how fit and healthy you feel.

-

You took control of yourself, and you are enjoying life.

-

You like to feel healthy and fit

-

Because your stomach is as small as a golf ball now. One bite and you feel full.

-

It's a part of you now.

-

You're in control of your eating habits.

-

The surgery was perfect, and you can finally feel proud of the change.

-

You're delighted with being healthy and fit.

-

Your quality of life has improved.

-

You have much more energy and enthusiasm.

-

You have much more control than many other aspects of your life...

-

Your self-esteem has become much more substantial.

-

With this image of you, you feel more attractive and pleasantly regarded.

-

You keep feeding yourself healthy

-

It is your new image

-

You feel and see your body clearly

You radiate confidence, and you're proud of yourself.

-

You did it; you achieved your goal. It is already a reality

-

I'll count again from 1 to 3. When I get to number 3, you will relax ten times more profoundly, focused, and determined to maintain your new food balance.

Let's start: 1...2...3...

-

You are ten times more focused

-

Your mind is receptive and calm

You feel a positive feeling spreading through your body.

-

You feel more determined than ever before.

-

Repeat after me: My stomach is the size of a golf ball.

-

Repeat after me: I eat the right amount of healthy, nutritious food.

-

Repeat after me: I like the taste of fresh, clear water.

-

Repeat after me: I exercise and stay fit

-

Repeat after me: I eat fruit and vegetables with pleasure.

-

Repeat after me: I feel full after a light, healthy meal.

.

These feelings take root sincerely in your mind and are your reality.

-

Your unconscious mind continues to see this positive outcome

-

You respond much better to lives' difficulties.

And you continue to feel more determined

-

Breathe deeply and slowly.

-

You are living with renewed confidence and courage. Your self-esteem grows more and more.

-

You are satisfied with your gastric band.

It doesn't take much to make you feel full.

-

You think more clearly and remain calm even in the most challenging situations, calmly developing greater inner strength.

-

You can concentrate your mind with confidence and get what you want.

-

In a few moments, I'll count from one to ten. With each number, you'll get more and more awake.

-

At number 8, you'll open your eyes, and at number 10, you'll be awake.

-

1.. 2.. 3.. Wake up.

-

4...5... - wake up...

-

6..7...8 open your eyes....

-

9 – 10

Now you're awake, and your diet is healthy and balanced and you can feel that band around your stomach.

CHAPTER 17:

Self-Hypnosis Techniques to Help You Stay on Track at Home

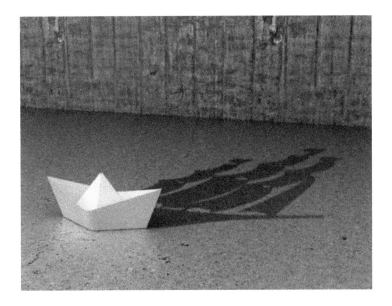

The only significant difference between hypnosis and self-hypnosis is that in the first one, the operator and the subject are two different people. In self-hypnosis, the operator and the issue coincide in the same person.

It is also a fact that learning is more comfortable and faster when done with another person.

The number of times it is necessary to reinforce the procedure depends entirely on you. If you practice the daily self-hypnosis exercise, one or two reinforcement sessions will be sufficient.

But what about those who have no one with whom to share the learning experience of self-hypnosis? What can they do? How can they learn?

Leave your worries aside.

It is possible to use self-hypnosis to solve virtually any type of problem and broaden your consciousness and connect with your innate superior intelligence and creative ability. By using self-hypnosis for the latter purpose, hypnosis can transform into meditation.

Self-hypnosis can also be used in those moments when you feel the need for a higher power to intervene in some situations; then it becomes a prayer. The subtle differences between these forms of self-hypnosis lie in the way thoughts are guided once the state of consciousness itself has altered, that is when the alpha state has reached.

Then I will tell you a fun experience that happened to me with self-hypnosis. I had an appointment with the dentist to have two molars removed. Last night I had conditioned myself to stop the flow of blood.

On the day of the appointment, when sitting in the dentist's chair, I self-reported. When the dentist removed the teeth, I blocked the flow of blood so that it did not flow through the open wound. The dentist was perplexed and kept telling his assistant: «It doesn't bleed.

How is it possible? I don't understand it. I smiled since I couldn't physically smile because of all the devices, cotton, and objects that held my mouth. Besides, I visualized quick and complete healing. After seventy-two hours the swelling had subsided, and the wounds had healed completely;

And now, I will tell you another funny experience that one of my patients had with self-hypnosis.

He was part of a group that participated in an investigation about dreams at the local hospital. Once a week, my patient slept in the hospital with an electroencephalogram (EEG) connected to his head. This was intended to record the waves of their brain activity.

By observing the graph, doctors could establish if they were an alpha, beta, tit, or delta, and they could also state when the patient was sleeping and when he was awake. My client immediately hypnotized himself as soon as he connected to the EEG.

The apparatus recorded a deep alpha state, indicative that the subject was sleeping, although he was fully awake. One of the doctors asked: "What's going on here?" Then the man alternately returned to the beta state, then to alpha, then again to beta, and finally to alpha while the machine registered it.

The changes confused the doctors until the subject told them what he was doing. The response of the doctors cannot reproduce here.

I have devised and written practically all the contents of this guidebook in an alpha state. What does this mean? It means that it is possible to develop an activity and keep your eyes open even if one is in an altered state of consciousness. Think about it for a moment.

It transports us to another state while we are comfortably and quietly sitting with our eyes closed, thinking about a specific objective. But using self-hypnosis in this sense is not easy to achieve since it requires a prolonged period of preconditioning in a hypnotic or auto hypnotic state. Such preconditioning is similar to that used for diet control, but the indications are different; It will be necessary to devise the techniques and suggestions for this case.

And it also requires practice, a lot of practice. Do not forget my words; time and effort will reward with the results. Develop your discipline and stick to it; The results will be a real success.

Guided Daily Meditation in Performing Self-Hypnosis

The experience of this guided meditation will be enhanced if you find yourself in a comfortable and ventilated spot.

Ensure that there is no disturbance from anything or anyone for thirty minutes.

At this particular moment, there is nothing that you need to worry about. You are at peace, and you are safe. You will allow the tensions of the day to dissipate so that you can connect with your inner self. With your eyes closes, breathe deeply and slowly through your nose and then exhale through your mouth. When you breathe in, you are taking all that is good and positive about this world into your body, and when you breathe, you are letting go of all tensions and unnecessary fears.

Now, inhale again. Breathe in slowly through your nose to the count of four.

One, two, three, and four.

With your lungs now full of oxygen, hold your breath for two seconds.

One and two.

And now exhale slowly through your mouth. You need to emit to the count of four.

One, two, three, and four.

When you breathe in, you can slowly feel your diaphragm expand when you feel the air enter your lungs. Breathe in until you feel like your lungs are full of air.

Strive to control the exhalation of air and make sure that you breathe out steadily

You need to continue this cycle of rhythmic breathing.

Inhale to the count for four.

Hold your breath for a count of two.

Exhale your breath to the count of four.

You can resume breathing normally, and you will feel all the tension in your body slowly dissipate.

Acknowledge that your body is now starting to feel more relaxed. Your arms and legs will begin to feel heavier.

Relax the tension in your lower back, middle-back, and your upper back. We often tend to store stress in our shoulders. Learn to release it. When you let go of the tension you feel in your body, you can contact your body relax.

Elongate your neck so that there is a space between your ears and shoulders. When you slowly elongate your neck, you can feel the mattress you are lying on or the chair that you are sitting on support your back.

Now, scan your body and check if there are any areas of tension left. If you feel that there are some, then you need to tighten the muscles in those areas and let go deliberately. Once you do this, you can contact your body to relax. You can feel the tension leaving your body.

Now, you need to go into a state of deep meditation.

To do this, you need to continue the rhythmic breathing exercise.

Imagine that you are now standing in a beautiful meadow with soft rays of sunlight falling on you.

You can see an arched doorway carved into a rising cliff.

Your surroundings look quite peaceful, and you feel good.

You can see golden sandy beaches behind you and azure blue skies above you.

Now, you are slowly making your way to the arched doorway. The door is within your reach; the wood feels warm under your fingers. As you trail your fingers across the door, you can feel a sense of excitement and wonder as you imagine what lies behind the door.

To enter, you need to keep your mind open to the wonders that lie ahead. Reach out and slowly turn the handle of the door.

As you emerge, you can see a lush and beautiful, bright-green rainforest.

A few moments ago, the air felt fresh and pleasant under the canopy and the welcome change from the sun-drenched beach.

Take a deep breath and then exhale to embrace this sense of peace.

As you start to walk forward, you notice a trail that leads through this beautiful rainforest.

As you look up, you can see glimpses of a beautiful blue sky speckled with soft, cotton-like clouds.

Continue scanning the sky all around you.

You are surrounded by majestic mahogany trees that reach up tall towards the zenith.

You marvel at the dark brown bark of the trees that seems to have a pleasantly sweet odor.

Space is limited here, but you are grateful for the narrow trail that leads you through this place of natural wonder.

You can listen to the melodious chirping of birds all around you.

It feels like the forest has come alive around you.

All of these appeals to your senses, and you can experience nature in its pristine form.

Consider if you strip back your own life and where to live more naturally, how much better you will feel.

Only a small percent of sunlight can penetrate onto the floor of this rainforest. So, you move further out in the wilderness; you can see the flashes of exotic blue butterflies dancing around you.

You can hear the melodic sound of running water in the distance and feel compelled to move towards it.

As you take in the wonder of the beautiful nature all around you, you move towards the more massive expanse of the forest area that leads to a delicate stream of water.

There are natural stepping-stones that lead you to a pool of water that looks crystal clear. Green plants surround the pool of water.

You walk closer to the pool, and you notice plants with colorful berries all around.

There are several fruit-bearing plants, and everything looks rich, exotic, and tempting.

You take a bite of these delicious berries, and you can feel a burst of flavors.

Start to concentrate on your breathing. Inhale as you open up your chest and exhale slowly.

It is time that you start to feel good about the person you are. It is time to feel content and embrace pure inner peace. Here in this rainforest, you are free to explore and be the person that you want to be.

Let go of any unhealthy eating habits; it is time to be kind to your body and to nurture and protect your body.

Repeat these affirmations to yourself and believe in each word.

Believe in the message and the power these words have to change your life.

I will change my perception of my body.

I recognize my self-worth.

I will change my eating habits so that I see my food as fuel and nutrients rather than comfort food.

I will exchange binge eating for breathing techniques and guided visualization.

I will start exercising and changing how I look and feel.

I will create an activity diary and plan on how to embrace exercise.

I am ready to face my inner fears and make the necessary positive changes.

Sit quietly for a moment and let these affirmations become a part of you.

It is time to feel positive about your life.

It is time to face any weight issues head-on.

You have the power to do so.

At any time, you can return to this rainforest and experience the wonders of nature. You can find your inner strength and inspiration in this haven.

You are centered, and you retain the feeling of peace and wonder.

Enjoy the moment and the feeling of harmony that you experience.

Breathe in and then out.

Retain your sense of peace and your desire to nurture your body.

Breathe in and out.

You will change your association with food.

Breathe in and out.

Slowly open your eyes on the count of three.

One, two, and three.

Now, you are back in your reality.

Stretch your body slowly and continue to take deep breaths.

Realize how good you feel in this moment.

Remember your desire to improve your fitness and your wellbeing.

Return to this haven of yours whenever you want to improve your health.

CHAPTER 18:

Why Is It Hard to Lose Weight?

For anyone who has ever struggled with weight, life can seem like an uphill battle. It can be downright devastating to see how difficult it can be to turn things around and shed some weight.

The fact of the matter is that losing weight doesn't have to be an uphill battle. Most of this requires you to understand better why this struggle happens and what you can do to help give yourself a fighting chance.

Physiological factors are affecting your ability to lose weight. There are also psychological, emotional, and even spiritual causes that affect your overall body's ability to help you lose weight and reach your ideal weight levels.

The Obvious Culprits

The obvious culprits that are holding you back are diet, a lack of exercise, and a combination of both.

First off, your diet plays a crucial role in your overall health and wellbeing. When it comes to weight management, your diet has everything to do with your ability to stay in shape and ward of unwanted weight.

When it comes to diet, we are not talking about keto, vegan, or Atkins; we are talking about the common foods which you consume and the amounts that you have of each one, which is why diet is one of the obvious culprits. If you have a diet that is high in fat, high in sodium, and high in sugar, you can rest assured that your body will end up gaining weight at a rapid rate.

When you consume high amounts of sugar, carbs, and fats, your body transforms them into glucose, which storing it in the body as fat. Of course, a proportion of the glucose produced by your body is used up as energy. However, if you consume far more than you need, your body isn't going to get rid of it; your body is going to hold on to it and make sure that it is stored for a rainy day.

Here is another vital aspect to consider: sweet and salty foods, the kind that we love so dearly, trigger "happy hormones" in the brain, namely dopamine. Dopamine is a hormone that is released by the body when it "feels good". And the food is one of the best ways to trigger it, which is why you somehow feel better after eating your favorite meals. It also explains the reason why we resort to food when we are not feeling well, which is called "comfort food", and it is one of the most popular coping mechanisms employed by folks around the world.

This rush of dopamine causes a person to become addicted to food. As with any addiction, there comes a time when you need to get more and more of that same substances to meet your body's requirements.

As a result of diet, a lack of regular exercise can do a number on your ability to lose weight and maintain a healthy balance. What regular exercise does is increase your body's overall caloric requirement. As such, your metabolism needs to convert fat at higher rates to keep up with your body's energy demands.

As the body's energetic requirements increase, that is, as your exercise regimen gets more and more intense, you will find that you will need increased amounts of both oxygen and glucose, which is one of the reasons why you feel hungrier when you ramp up your workouts.

However, increased caloric intake isn't just about consuming more and more calories for the sake of consuming more and more calories; you need to consume an equal amount of proteins, carbs, fats, and vitamins too for your body to build the necessary elements that will build muscle, foster movement and provide proper oxygenation in the blood.

Moreover, nutrients are required for the body to recover. One of the byproducts of exercise is called "lactic acid". Lactic acid builds up in the muscles as they get more and more tired. Lactic acid signals the body that it is time to stop working out or risk injury if you continue. Without lactic acid, your body would have no way of knowing when your muscles have overextended their capacity.

After you have completed your workout, the body needs to get rid of the lactic acid buildup. So, if you don't have enough of the right minerals in your body, for example, potassium, your muscles will ache for days until your body is finally able to get rid of the lactic acid buildup. This example goes to show how proper nutrition is needed to help the body get moving and also recover once it is done exercising.

As a result, a lack of exercise reconfigures your body's metabolism to work at a slower pace. What that means is that you need to consume fewer calories to fuel your body's lack of exercise. So, if you end up wasting more than you need, your body will just put it away for a rainy day. Plain and simple.

The Sneaky Culprits

The sneaky culprits are the ones that aren't quite so overt in causing you to gain weight or have trouble shedding pounds. These culprits hide beneath the surface but are very useful when it comes to keeping you overweight. The first culprit we are going to be looking at is called "stress".

Stress is a potent force. From an evolutionary perspective, it exists as a means of fueling the flight-or-fight response. Stress is the human response to danger. When a person senses danger, the body begins to secrete a hormone called "cortisol". When cortisol begins running through the body, it signals the entire system to prep for a potential showdown. Depending on the situation, it might be best to hightail it out and live to fight another day.

In our modern way of life, stress isn't so much a response to life and death situations (though it can certainly be). Instead, it is the response to cases that are deemed as "conflictive" by the mind. This could be a confrontation with a co-worker, bumper to bumper traffic, or any other type of situation in which a person feels vulnerable in some way.

Throughout our lives, we subject to countless interactions in which we must deal with stress. In general terms, the feelings of alertness subside when the perceived threat is gone. However, when a person is exposed to prolonged periods of stress, any number of changes can happen.

One such change is overexposure to cortisol. When there is too much cortisol in the body, the body's overall response is to hoard calories, increase the production of other hormones such as adrenaline and kick up the immune system's function.

This response by the body is akin to the panic response that the body would assume when faced with prolonged periods of hunger or fasting. As a result, the body needs to go into survival mode. Please bear in mind that the body has no clue if it is being chased by a bear, dealing with a natural disaster, or just having a bad day at the office. Regardless of the circumstances, the body is faced with the need to ensure its survival. So, anything that it eats goes straight to fat stores.

Moreover, a person's stressful situation makes them search for comfort and solace. There are various means of achieving this. Food is one of them. So is alcohol consumption. These two types of pleasures lead to significant use of calories. Again, when the body is in high gear, it will store as many calories and keep them in reserve.

This what makes you gain weight when you are stressed out.

Another of the sneaky culprits is sleep deprivation. In short, sleep deprivation is sleeping less than the recommended 8 hours that all adults should sleep. In the case of children, the recommended amount of sleep can be anywhere from 8 to 12 hours, depending on their age.

Granted, some adults can function perfectly well with less than 8 hours' sleep. Some folks can work perfectly well with 6 hours' sleep, while there are folks who are shattered when they don't get eight or even more hours' sleep. This is different for everyone as each individual is different in this regard.

That being said, sleep deprivation can trigger massive amounts of cortisol. This, fueled by ongoing exposure to stress, leads the body to further deepening its panic mode. When this occurs, you can rest assured that striking a healthy balance between emotional wellbeing and physical health can be nearly impossible to achieve.

Now, the best way to overcome sleep deprivation is to get sleep. But that is easier said than done. One of the best ways to get back on track to a certain degree is to get in enough sleep when you can.

The last sneaky culprit on our list is emotional distress. Emotional distress can occur as a result of any number of factors. For example, the loss of a loved one, a stressful move, a divorce, or the loss of a job can all contribute to large amounts of emotional distress. While all of the situations mentioned above begin as a stressful situation, they can fester and lead to severe psychological issues. Over time, these emotional issues can grow into more profound topics such as General Anxiety Disorder or Depression. Studies have shown that prolonged periods of stress can lead to depression and a condition known as Major Depression.

The most common course of treatment for anxiety and depression is the use of an antidepressant. And guess what: one of the side effects associated with antidepressants is weight. The reason for this is that antidepressants tinker with the brain's chemistry in such a way that they alter the brain's processing of chemicals through the suppression of serotonin transport. This causes the brain to readjust its overall chemistry. Thus, you might find the body unable to process food quite the same way. In general, it is common to see folks gain as much as 10 pounds as a result of taking antidepressants.

As you can see, weight gain is not the result of "laziness" or being "undisciplined". Sure, you might have to clean up your diet somewhat and get more exercise. But the causes we have outlined here ought to provide you with enough material to see why there are less obvious causes that are keeping you from achieving your ideal weight. This is why meditation plays such a key role in helping you deal with stress and emotional strife while helping you find a balance between your overall mental and physical wellbeing.

Ultimately, the strategies and techniques that we will further outline here will provide you with the tools that will help you strike that balance and eventually lead you to find the most effective way in which you will deal with the rigors of your day to day life while being able to make the most out of your efforts to lead a healthier life. You have everything you need to do it. So, let's find out how you can achieve this.

CHAPTER 19:

Weight Loss Tips to Practice Every Day

Keeping up a contemporary, quick-paced way of life can leave a brief period to oblige your necessities. You are moving always starting with one thing then onto the next, not focusing on what your psyche or body truly needs. Rehearsing mindfulness can help you to comprehend those necessities.

When eating mindfulness is connected, it can help you recognize your examples and practices while simultaneously standing out to appetite and completion related to body signs.

Originating from the act of pressure decrease dependent on mindfulness, rehearsing mindfulness while eating can help you focus on the present minute instead of proceeding with ongoing and unacceptable propensities.

Individuals that need to be cautious about sustenance and nourishment are asked to:

➤ Explore their inward knowledge about sustenance—different preferences

➤ Choose sustenance that pleases and support their bodies

➤ Accept explicit sustenance inclinations without judgment or self-analysis

➤ Practice familiarity with the indications of their bodies beginning to eat and quit eating.

The Most Effective Method to Start Eating More Intentionally

Stage 1: Eat Before You Shop. We have all been there. You go with a rumbling stomach to the shop. You meander the passageways, and out of the blue, those power bars and microwaveable suppers start to look truly enticing. "When you're excessively ravenous, shopping will, in general, shut us off from our progressively talented goals of eating in a way that searches useful for the body," says Dr. Rossy. So, even if you feel the slightest craving or urge to eat, get a nutritious bite or a light meal before heading out. That way, your food choices will be made intentionally when you shop, as opposed to propelled by craving or an unexpected sugar crash in the blood.

Stage 2: Make Conscious Food Choices. When you truly start considering where your nourishment originates from, you're bound to pick sustenance that is better for you, the earth, and the people occupied with the expanding procedure portrays Meredith Klein, an astute cooking educator, and Pranaful's author. "When you're in the supermarket, focus on the nourishment source," Klein shows. "Hope to check whether it's something that has been created in this country or abroad and endeavors to know about pesticides that may have been exposed to or presented to people who were developing nourishment." If you can, make successive adventures to your neighborhood ranchers advertise, where most sustenance is developed locally, she recommends.

Stage 3: Enjoy the Preparation Process. "When you get ready sustenance, instead of looking at it as an errand or something you need to hustle through, value the process. You can take a great deal of pleasure in food shopping for items that you know will help you feel better and nourish your body.

Stage 4: "Simply eat". This is something we once in a while do, as simple as it sounds, "simply eat." "Individuals regularly eat while doing different things — taking a gander at their telephones, TVs, PCs, and books, and mingling," claims Dr. Rossy. "While cautious eating can happen when you're doing other stuff, endeavor to' simply eat' at whatever point plausible." She includes that centering the nourishment you're eating without preoccupation can make you mindful of flavors you may never have taken note of. Yum!

Stage 5: Down Your Utensils. When you are done eating, immediately put your dishes and utensils away. This is a way of signaling to yourself that you are done eating (it tends to be much a bit tough to accept). "You're getting a charge out of each chomp that way, and you're focused on the nibble that is in your mouth right now as opposed to setting up the following one," Klein says.

Stage 6: Chew, Chew, Chew Your Food. Biting your sustenance is exceptionally fundamental and not only for, you know, not to stun. "When we cautiously eat our sustenance, we help the body digest the nourishment all the more effectively and meet a greater amount of our dietary needs," says Dr. Rossy. Furthermore, no, we won't educate you how often you've eaten your sustenance. However, Dr. Rossy demonstrates biting until the nourishment is very much separated – which will most likely take more than a couple of quick eats.

Stage 7: Check-In with Your Hunger. You frequently miss the sign that your body sends you during supper when you eat thoughtlessly, for example, when supper time turns into your prime time to make up for lost time with Netflix appears or when you have your supper in a rush. At the end of the day, the one that illuminates you when you begin to feel total. Dr. Rossy proposes ending dinner and taking some time with your craving levels to check-in. "Keep eating in case no doubt about it," she proposes. "In case you're not ravenous yet, spare the nourishment for some other time, manure it, or even discard it." Those remains can make the following day an incredible dinner of care.

Last but not least, we get it; life does not always allow sit-down, completely tuned-in mealtimes. So, if you don't have time for all seven steps, attempt to include one or two in each dinner. "If you have only a little window of time, just try to devote yourself to food," suggests Klein. "Set down your phone, get away from the screen, just be there–you can do that regardless of how much time you have."

Tips in Mindful Eating that Transform how you Relate to Food

We lose ourselves in regular daily existence designs each day. Our propensity for vitality pushes and pulls us to and from, and we are left with minimal opportunity to encounter life in a way that, for this very time, we are completely present.

Sometime in the not so distant future, to-day tasks get more from this autopilot state than others. There are a few things we do so regularly in our lives that we become like automatons, doing them all day every day thoughtlessly and commonly. These exercises incorporate strolling, driving, specific sorts of occupation, and eating.

Yet, these exercises additionally loan themselves to the activity of care, because while these examples are speaking to the draw of propensity vitality, they are likewise the perfect thing to snatch on when in any predefined time we need to turn out to be completely present in our life.

Consideration is both the quality and the activity of getting to be completely present at this very time in our life. It's mindfulness that empowers us to break these standard examples and make a move for a progressively alert and present life.

Eating might be more than whatever another movement that fits the activity of cognizance. This because we discover the flavors we experience when we frequently devour fascinating and various, just as the pleasurable demonstration of eating. Thus, it is through the simple exercise of careful gobbling that we can wake up to our life and discover more harmony and joy all the while.

On occasion, we can likewise identify poor practices with nourishment and eating. These poor propensities can cause us a ton of torment, some even respected issue.

The act of eating mindfully can spark a light on our standard eating and sustenance related propensities. What's more, in doing such, we can ease a lot of the agony on our plate identified with the nourishment.

- **Simply eat mindfully.** Take a minute before eating to see the nourishment's smell, visual intrigue, and even surface. Appreciate the various vibes that go with your feast. This concise minute will help open up your cognizance with the goal that you become all the more completely dynamic in the eating demonstration.

- **Take your time**. Remember to lift your hand/fork/spoon and bite the sustenance itself. Give close consideration to each flavor in your mouth and notice how the nourishment you eat feels and scents. Be completely present for the biting go about as your central matter of (light) focus during cautious eating.

- **Recognize thoughts, feelings, and sensations.** When in your general vicinity of awareness, thoughts, feelings, or different sensations emerge, just be aware of them, recognize their reality, and after that, let them go as though they were gliding on a cloud.

CHAPTER 20:

Hypnotic Meditation to Lose Weight

[Notes for the speaker are marked in brackets. This text should be read slowly, with plenty of pauses to allow rest and time for the words to sink into the listener, time for them to become sleepy. Significant pauses have been marked within the text.]

Welcome.

This meditation will guide you into a deep state of relaxation. From that place of peace, you will effortlessly absorb positive affirmations that will help you to lose weight with ease.

Repeat this meditation practice regularly. All you have to do is listen — don't worry about making a conscious effort to sit in formal meditation. Don't feel that you need to solve any problems or come to any great realizations while you listen. And don't worry about whether you're 'doing it right'.

By listening, you are doing it right. You are prioritizing your health. You are showing concern for your sense of calm. You are increasing your innate ability to understand the physical needs of your body.

By simply listening, you are sending a message of self-respect to your subconscious; and every time you repeat the meditation, your subconscious receives that message again. Each time, the message becomes stronger.

And this repetition creates neurological pathways in your brain that make it easier and easier for you to access the power of the positive affirmations you'll work with during this meditation.

[Pause]

Now, start by getting comfortable. Towards the end of this practice, you will start to feel blissfully sleepy, and you'll begin to drift into a deep, peaceful sleep. So, make sure that you're lying down somewhere cozy and safe, where you can happily rest.

Ideally, it's the evening, and you're ready to go to bed for the night. You're in bed. You're a comfortable temperature — if you feel too hot or too cold, then make any adjustments you need to make now; perhaps adding or removing layers of clothing or blankets or turning the heating up or down.

Then lie on your back. Allow your feet to drop out to the side; your legs are relaxed. Rest your right hand on your lower abdomen, and your left hand on your chest.

For the next 90 seconds, bring your awareness to your breath. Don't try to control it or change it; just notice the breath.

Notice the length and depth of the breath. The coolness of the air as it enters at the tip of the nose, and the warmer air leaving your body. Notice whether the breath fills your belly, or your ribcage, or stays even higher up in the chest. And notice the quality of the breath — is it easy? Smooth? Raspy? Does it catch or falter?

There is no right or wrong. Notice the natural rhythm of your breath.

Thoughts will come into your mind — that's fine. Allow the thoughts to come. There's no need to judge them. Let them sit in your mind for a moment, and then gently bring the awareness back to the breath.

[90 second pause]

Good. Now, we'll spend some time using the breath to calm the nervous system and move into a state of deeper relaxation. Learning to harness the power of the breath is incredibly valuable, and it can help you to make positive changes in your habitual ways of living. By cultivating awareness of breath and learning how to deepen and direct the breath, you also cultivate awareness of the whole body.

As this awareness develops, your natural intuition becomes stronger. You become more able to recognize the kinds of food that feel good and nourishing and healthy for your body — the food that can support you in living the energetic and active lifestyle that you want. When you can feel food doing wonderful things for your body, you start to crave that food. Without having to force yourself and without feeling as though you're depriving yourself of anything, you'll start to eat more vegetables and fruits, more lean proteins, and more whole grains.

And you become more in tune to feeling the benefits of exercise. When you can feel how a period of exercise has brought you to life — when you can feel how much stronger your heart feels, and how much more free your lungs feel, and how much extra energy and focus you possess as you glide through the day — then you'll want to exercise. Not because you feel like you should. But because it makes you feel good.

So, before we start to work with the breath, here is your first of three affirmations to help you lose weight and improve your health:

I am going to eat more healthy food because I deserve to feel good.

You do deserve to feel good. Repeat this affirmation three times with me. If you feel comfortable doing so, you could speak them out loud. If not, repeat them silently in your mind. Affirmations are just as powerful when you repeat them silently; what's important is that you focus on them fully.

Remember how you were consciously aware of the natural rhythm of your breath a few minutes ago? Bring that same conscious awareness to this affirmation. Now:

I am going to eat more healthy food because I deserve to feel good.

I am going to eat more healthy food because I deserve to feel good.

I am going to eat more healthy food because I deserve to feel good.

[Pause]

Great. Bring the awareness back to the breath. Take a few easy, natural breaths.

Your right hand is still on your lower abdomen; your left hand on your chest.

With the next inhale, start to breathe into the right hand. The right hand rises with the breath as the belly is blown up like a balloon. Fill the abdomen as much as you can, and then when you can't breathe into the belly anymore, start to exhale. Gently allow the belly to fall; the right hand falls with it.

Again, take a deep, full abdominal breath. The right hand rests on the lower abdomen, so it rises as you inhale and falls slowly as you exhale slowly.

Take three more breaths like this.

Into the right hand.

Out of the right hand.

Into the right hand.

Out of the right hand.

Into the right hand.

Out of the right hand.

Well done. Let go of control of the breath — again, take a couple of easy, natural breaths.

[Pause]

And then we'll start to breathe into the left hand.

With the next inhale, start to fill the chest with air. The chest rises as much as possible — all the way up to the collarbone. The left hand rises as the chest rises. The shoulders may move up slightly.

And when you can't inhale any more air into the chest, start to breathe out. Allow the chest to fall; start at the top, so the collarbone falls first, and then the middle of the chest, and then the ribs fall. The left hand falls with the chest.

Really good. And again: another deep, full breath into the chest. The abdomen stays still — it doesn't rise as you breathe into the chest. And exhale slowly.

Take three more breaths like this.

Into the left hand.

Out of the left hand.

Into the left hand.

Out of the left hand.

Into the left hand.

Out of the left hand.

And then let go of control of the breath and take a few easy, undirected breaths.

[Pause]

Now we'll combine the right hand and the left hand to create a full, deep pattern of breath. This breathing technique works with the full motion of the diaphragm — the big muscle behind your ribcage, which helps your body to control and direct the breath.

Breathing like this has an almost instant effect on the nervous system. It signals to the brain that all is well; there's nothing to worry about, and allows the parasympathetic nervous system to lead. This mechanism of the nervous system gives your body a chance to rest and heal; to digest food, and to restore energy.

This kind of deep, diaphragmatic breath also tones the muscles of the abdominal wall and gently massages the internal organs. So not only does it help you relax, but it also helps you to develop muscle strength and internal wellbeing.

When you've got the hang of this breathing technique, you can repeat your second affirmation with each breath. Your second affirmation is:

I am going to move my body in ways that I enjoy because I deserve to feel good.

[Pause]

Let's begin.

First, breathe into the right hand. The belly rises. When the belly can't rise any more, start to breathe into the left hand. Chest rises. All the way to the collarbone.

And then breathe out of the left hand — so the chest begins to fall first. And then breathe out of the right hand, so the belly falls. Allow the body to soften with that wonderful long exhale.

Great. Now, take a second deep, full breath. Inhale into the right hand; and then into the left hand. All the way up to the collarbone.

Exhale out of the left hand; chest falls. And out of the right hand, belly falls. Enjoy that feeling of softening.

Take three more breaths like this.

Into the right hand; left hand.

Out of the left hand; right hand.

Into the right hand; left hand.

Out of the left hand; right hand.

Into the right hand; left hand.

Out of the left hand; right hand.

Perfect. Now you can start to use your second affirmation.

As you inhale, repeat the first part of the affirmation:

I am going to move my body in ways that I enjoy…

And on the exhale, repeat the second part:

because I deserve to feel good.

Breathe slowly and think the words slowly.

When you're ready, let's do it together five times.

Inhale into the right hand, then the left hand, and repeat:

I am going to move my body in ways that I enjoy…

Exhale out of the left hand, then the right hand, and repeat:

because I deserve to feel good.

Inhale: I am going to move my body in ways that I enjoy…

Exhale: because I deserve to feel good.

Inhale: I am going to move my body in ways that I enjoy…

Exhale: because I deserve to feel good.

Inhale: I am going to move my body in ways that I enjoy…

Exhale: because I deserve to feel good.

Inhale: I am going to move my body in ways that I enjoy…

Exhale: because I deserve to feel good.

And relax. Allow the breath to return to a natural rhythm. No effort in the body at all.

[Pause]

Well done. There is no more physical work to do. Your breathing practice has soothed your nervous system. Your body is calming down and finding its rest state. A state of deep relaxation. A state of complete ease.

Take a moment to enjoy this gentle shift from an active body to a restful body.

[Pause]

Notice the mind beginning to rest as the body rests.

You are moving closer to a deep and peaceful sleep. A wonderfully healing rest. As your nervous system relaxes, your body is already beginning to rebuild cells; to restore wellness. The energy that you've used today is being replenished and renewed.

All of this is already happening.

It takes no conscious work. Your body knows how to do this. All you have to do is be. It is effortless.

Your body knows how to carry you into sleep if you release control and allow it to happen.

You don't need to read books or get a nutritionist's advice to become healthier. You have all the knowledge you need within the systems of your body. The key is listening.

CHAPTER 21:

Positive Impacts of Affirmations

Y ou control the fundamental fixings that make self-hypnosis work for you. These are similar fixings that make your experience of achievement for any objective you pick. Let us take a gander at every component and how you may utilize it to perform for you.

Motivation

Motivation is the vitality of your craving, of what you need. Needing is an inclination that you can control. For the greater part of your life, you have chiefly controlled your craving or needing by restricting it or denying it. You might be truly adept at controlling your wants and needing in certain regions and powerless or natural in others. Since this is a "diet" book, you may have just set yourself up to hear that this "diet" will resemble the others that have mentioned to you what you should deny yourself or breaking point. That is, different diets have mentioned to you what not to need, and the accentuation may have been about "not needing" a few nourishments that you have developed to cherish. Welcome to another method of treating yourself; we will urge you to show signs of improvement at "needing." Denial is excluded from Rapid Weight Loss Hypnosis.

Your motivation is a key factor, one of the fundamental fixings. We need you to center your vitality of needing not toward food yet toward the motivation that unmistakably tells your mind-body what you need it to make: flawless weight. We urge you to get great at needing your ideal weight. Here is a model. Let us state that you are in a pool, and out of nowhere, you take in a significant piece of water. At that time, you need just a single thing, a breath of air. It feels decisive, and a breath of air is the main thing on your mind as of now. The needing is so serious and powerful that it dominates every single other idea and urges you to take the necessary steps to get that breath of air. That is the amount we need you to need the weight and self perception that you want.

Conviction and Believing

Convictions are those musings and thoughts that are valid for you. They don't need to be deductively demonstrated for you to realize that they generally will be valid for you. Insite that, you know about it or not, your activities, both mindful and subconscious, depend on your convictions. Even though your convictions are contemplations and thoughts, they shape your experience by influencing your activities throughout everyday life. If you accept that creatures make great sidekicks, you most likely have a feline or canine or parrot or a ferret or two. If you accept that espresso keeps you alert around evening time, you likely don't drink espresso before hitting the sack. The power of accepting lets you impact your body in manners that may appear to be bewildering. Fake treatment reactions, where people react to an inactive substance as though it were genuine medicine, are regular instances of how convictions are knowledgeable about the body. If an individual truly accepts that he will get well when taking specific medicine, it will happen whether the tablet contains a prescription or is inactive. Similarly, if an individual truly accepts that he can accomplish high evaluations in school, it will occur. If an individual truly accepts that he can achieve his ideal weight, it will occur.

Recollect your pretend games as a kid. Your capacity to imagine is similarly as solid now as when you were exceptionally youthful. It might be somewhat corroded, and you may require a touch of training, yet when you permit yourself to imagine and let yourself have faith in what you are imagining, you will find a powerful apparatus. You will find this is a brilliantly viable approach to convey your goals, those messages of what you need, to the entirety of the phones and tissues and organs of your body, which react by bringing that goal into reality for you. We can't state this enough: musings are things. The musings, the photos, the thoughts you put in your mind become the messages your self-hypnosis passes on to your mind-body, eventually transforming your ideal body into reality and imagining is picking what to accept and getting retained in those thoughts. Similarly, as an amplifying glass can center beams of daylight, you can center your psychological vitality to make your considerations, thoughts, and convictions genuine for your body.

Desire

You may not generally get what you need, yet you do get what you anticipate. Desires contain the vitality of convictions and become the aftereffects of what is accepted. Here is a case of how to "anticipate." When you plunked to peruse this book, you didn't analyze the seat or couch to test its capacity to hold your weight. You just plunked without contemplating it. You didn't need to consider it, because a piece of you is sure, and has such a great amount of confidence in the seat, that you simply "anticipated" it to hold you. That is the way to expect the ideal body weight you want. Remembering this, be mindful of what you state to yourself as well as other people concerning your body weight desires. "I generally put on weight over the special seasons."

Mind-Body in Focus

Every one of the fundamental fixings can create powerful outcomes when centered inside the mind-body. Nonetheless, when these fixings are adjusted appropriately inside the procedure of self-hypnosis, their viability has amplified a hundredfold. Self-hypnosis is a procedure for creating your world. You may think this sounds mystical or unrealistic. However, that is comparative with what you have encountered as yet in your life. These thoughts might be exceptionally new to you. Here is a case of the "relative" idea of new thoughts. Envision that you are given a personal jet that is flawlessly equipped with sumptuous arrangements and a very much prepared team. It is a brilliant blessing, and you get the opportunity to show this designing wonder to certain people who have seen nothing like it.

Your subconscious (mind-body) utilizes the mix of what you need (motivation), what you accept, and what you expect as a plan for activity. The outcomes are accomplished by your mind-body (subconscious) and not by deduction or breaking down. If an individual contact a virus surface that she accepts is hot, she can create a rankle or consume reaction. Then again, an individual contacting an extremely hot surface reasoning that it is cool may not deliver a consume reaction. Individuals who stroll over hot coals while envisioning that they are cool may encounter a warm physical issue (some minor singing on the bottoms of their feet). Yet, their invulnerable framework doesn't react with a consume (rankling, torment, and so on.) Because their minds advise their bodies how to respond. Once more, it is the arrangement of every one of the three of the basic fixings that make this conceivable:

• Wanting to do it

• Believing it conceivable

• Expecting to be fruitful

This is the way to progress. Your body completes your convictions. Your convictions direct your activities, which like this, shape your experience.

Some portray this procedure as creating your prosperity or creating your involvement with life. In our way of life, we see this depicted inside the motivational and positive mental disposition writing. It very well may be seen in numerous zones of mysticism. You can likewise think back to the people of yore and see it depicted in the provisions of the authentic period. An individual a lot smarter than we are stated, "It will be done unto you as per your conviction." In the current period of

EXTREME WEIGHT LOSS HYPNOSIS

integrative medication and brain research, we call it self-hypnosis or mind-body medication. There are currently various logical examinations that exhibit astonishing outcomes for torment control, wound mending, physical modification, and a lot of more medical advantages than we recently suspected conceivable.

Picking Your Beliefs

You can pick your convictions. You may decide to accept what you see, in the feeling of "See it to trust it" or "Truth can be stranger than fiction." This is simple to do. You experience something with your faculties, and that is a natural method of picking whether it is reasonable or not. However, you may likewise decide to trust it first and afterward observe it, which may require some training. The vast majority think that it's simpler to let the world mention to them what is valid or what to accept. The TV, media, papers, books, instructors, and specialists besiege us with what to accept. You grew up finding out about the world and yourself from numerous outside sources. This prompted a recognizable example of watching and accepting data about the world from outside yourself, and you picked which data to make a piece of your conviction framework. This included convictions about your body. For instance, when your stomach makes a thundering sound, you accept that it implies you are ravenous. Or then again, you feel queasy and trust you are wiped out. Both of these are instances of watched occasions: you watched an association once and decided to trust it.

In Rapid Weight Loss Hypnosis, we are suggesting that you turn that training around with this thought: "Trust it, and you will see it." This implies you initially pick what to accept, and afterward, your body follows up on it as evidence and makes it genuine, you would say. One of the significant messages we trust you will get from this book is that your mind-body hears all that you hear, all that you state, all that you think, picture, or envision in your mind, and it can't differentiate between what is genuine and what you envision. It follows up on what you need and anticipate. In light of this, which of these announcements would assist you with encountering the ideal weight you want: "I simply take a gander at food and put on weight" or "I can eat anything, and my weight remains the equivalent"? The last mentioned. In any case, which articulation do you by and by accept to be valid for you? Once more, it will be done unto you as indicated by your conviction. We will assist you with the thoughts, language, and pictures that plan compelling hypnotic proposals, yet you have all-out command over what you decide to accept.

As you read the thoughts of this book and hear the hypnotic recommendations offered during the trancework on the sound, you will settle on numerous decisions for yourself. We wholeheartedly urge you to decide to trust it so you will see it for yourself. Your subconscious (mind-body) can't differentiate and will follow up on what you select in any case. Why not select what you truly need?

The Energy of Emotions

Not all considerations and convictions show themselves in your experience. Just those that have the vitality of your sentiments (feelings), alongside your conviction and your desire that something will occur, will show themselves. Your sentiments or feelings are a type of vitality that impacts this procedure of creation.

CHAPTER 22:

Increase Your Wellbeing
with 100 Positive Affirmations

1. I am healthy, wealthy, and clever

2. I let go of the illness, I am not ill

3. Thanks to my creator and everyone in my life.

4. I am grateful for all the bounty that I already enjoy

5. Every day I grow energetically and vibrantly

6. I only give my body the necessary nutritious food

7. My body is my temple

8. You can always maintain a healthy weight

9. I deserve to enjoy perfect health

10. Act to be healthy

11. I respect my body and am willing to exercise

12. Affirmation for Rapid and Natural Weight Loss

13. My body is beautiful and healthy

14. I choose healthy and nutritious foods

15. I like to exercise, and I do it frequently

16. Losing weight is easy and even fun

17. I have confidence in myself

18. I am now sure of myself

19. I feel confident to succeed

20. From day to day, I am more and more confident

21. I am sure to reach my goal

22. I want to be a noble example

23. I believe in my value

24. I have the strength to realize my dreams

25. I am really adorable

26. I trust my inner wisdom

27. Everything I do satisfies me deeply

28. I trust the process of life

29. I can free the past and forgive

30. No thought of the past limits me

31. I get ready to change and grow

32. I am safe in the Universe, and life loves me and supports me

33. With joy, I observe how life supports me abundantly and provides me with more goods than I can imagine.

34. Freedom is my divine right

35. I accept myself and create peace in my mind and my heart

36. I am a loved person, and I am safe.

37. Divine Intelligence continually guides me in achieving my goals

38. I feel happy to live

39. I create peace in my mind, and my body reflects it with perfect health

40. All my experiences are opportunities to learn and grow

41. I flow with life easily and effortlessly

42. My ability to create the good in my life is unlimited

43. I deserve to be loved because I exist

44. I am a being worthy of love

45. I dare to try, and I'm proud of it

46. I choose to really love myself

47. I love myself and accept myself completely

48. I am ready to try new things

49. There are things I can already do, I just need to start even though I'm not ready yet

50. I am much more capable than I think

51. As I love myself, I allow others to love me too ...

52. I accumulate more and more confidence in myself

53. I am unique and perfect as I am

54. I am wonderful

55. I'm proud of everything I've accomplished

56. I do not have to be perfect, I just need to be myself

57. I feel able to succeed

58. I give myself permission to go out of my role as a victim and take more responsibility for my life

59. The past is over, I now have control of my life, and I move

60. I am my best friend

61. I am able to say "no" without fear of displeasing

62. I choose to clean myself of my fears and my doubts

63. Fear is a simple emotion that cannot stop me from succeeding

64. Every step forward I make increases my strength

65. My hesitations give way to victory

66. I want to do it, I can do it

67. I am capable of great things

68. There is no one more important than me

69. I may be wrong but that I can handle it

70. With confidence, I can accomplish everything

71. I allow myself to have a lot of fun

72. I deserve to be seen, heard, and shine

73. I deserve love and respect

74. I choose to believe in myself

75. I allow myself to feel good about myself and trust myself

76. I reduce measures quickly and easily

77. I can maintain my ideal weight without many problems

78. My body feels light and in perfect health

79. I'm motivated to lose weight and stay

80. Every day I reduce measures and lose weight

81. I fulfill my weight loss goals

82. I lose weight every day, and I recover my perfect figure

83. I eat like a thin person

84. I treat my body with love and give it healthy food

85. I choose to feel good inside and out

86. I feed myself only until I am satisfied, I don't saturate my food body

87. I know how to choose my food in a balanced way.

88. I feed slowly and enjoy every bite.

89. I am the only one who can choose how I eat and how I want to see myself.

90. It is easy for me to control the amount of what I eat.

91. I learn to have habits that lead me to my ideal weight.

92. Being at my ideal weight makes me feel healthy and young.

93. My body is very grateful and quickly reflects all the care I have with him.

94. My body reflects my perfect health.

95. I feel better every day

96. Being at my ideal weight motivates me to do other things that I like.

97. The human body is moldable, and I am the artist of my body.

98. Every day I eat with awareness.

99. I consume the calories needed to have an ideal weight and a healthy body.

100.   Every day I like the way I feel.

CHAPTER 23:

Deep Sleep for Weight Loss

There are several things you know you should follow when you are aiming to lose that extra weight. You eliminate junk foods and sugar from your diet and include lots of complex carbohydrates, lean proteins, and vegetables. You try to exercise as much as you can throughout the day and go to the gym regularly. However, what you don't realize is that one of the essential parts of losing weight is getting adequate sleep.

The Daily Express had reported that good sleep is the best recipe to reduce weight. It also said that people who can decrease their stress levels and get about 8 hours of sleep every night could double their weight loss. It's true: getting enough sleep can help you lose weight.

How Does Sleep Benefit Weight Loss?

The amount of sleep you can get becomes as essential as exercise and diet when you are trying to lose weight. Here are some reasons why sleeping properly can help you in losing weight:

· Inadequate amount of sleep tends to increase your appetite – Several studies have shown that people who get an inadequate amount of sleep have an increased appetite. This might be caused by the impact of sleep on the hormone leptin and ghrelin. These are 2 of the essential hunger hormones present in the human body. The hormone ghrelin, which is released in your stomach, signals to your brain that you're hungry. When your stomach is empty before you start eating, the level of ghrelin increases, while it decreases after you consume. The other hunger hormone leptin is released from fat cells. This hormone signals fullness to your brain and suppresses your hunger. In the absence of adequate sleep, your body reduces the production of leptin while increasing the ghrelin production, thus increasing your appetite and making you hungry.

· Inadequate sleep is a significant risk factor for obesity and weight gain – Shortage of sleep has been linked with weight gain and a higher BMI. Studies have shown that although people have different sleep requirements when they get less than 7 hours of sleep every night, it can cause weight changes. Moreover, several sleep disorders, such as sleep apnea, get worse due to weight gain. Therefore, a shortage of sleep can result in weight gain, which worsens sleep quality.

· Sleep helps prevent resistance to insulin – Your cells can become resistant to insulin because of poor sleep. The hormone insulin transports sugar from your blood into your body's cells so that your body can use it in the form of energy. However, if your cells become resistant to insulin, the sugar fails to enter the cells and remains in your bloodstream. To compensate for this, more insulin is produced by your body, which ends up making you feel hungrier. As a result, your body stores the extra calories as fat. Resistance to insulin can cause both weight gain and type-2 diabetes.

· Sleep helps you make healthy choices by fighting cravings – Sleep deprivation can change the way your brain works,

making it more difficult for you to resist cravings and make healthy choices. Lack of sleep dulls the activity of your brain's frontal lobe, which makes decisions and controls impulses. Moreover, when you're sleep-deprived, the reward centers of your brain get more stimulated by food. Studies also suggest that inadequate sleep can increase your affinity for high-calorie foods.

· Inadequate sleep can reduce your resting metabolism – The number of calories burnt by your body when you are at rest is known as your resting metabolic rate or RMR. Studies reveal that lack of sleep can decrease your RMR. In one study where fifteen men were kept awake for twenty-four hours, their resting metabolic rate found to be five percent less than usual, and their metabolic rate was after consuming food was found to be twenty percent lower. Moreover, lack of sleep can also result in muscle loss.

· Sleep can increase physical activity – Poor sleep can result in daytime fatigue, which can decrease your motivation to exercise. Moreover, it's more likely that you will get tired quickly while applying. A study done on fifteen people revealed that when the participants were deprived of sleep, the intensity and amount of their physical exercise reduced. Thus, getting an adequate amount of proper sleep can help improve your athletic performance.

Therefore, to maintain your weight, you must get quality sleep along with the right diet and exercise. The way your body responds to food can dramatically be altered by inadequate sleep. For starters, as your appetite grows, it will become difficult for you to resist temptations and control your portion size. This turns into a vicious cycle. A shortage of sleep will make you gain weight, and it will make it harder for you to get adequate sleep. However, following healthy sleeping habits can help you lose weight and maintain a healthy body.

CHAPTER 24:

Gastric Band Hypnosis for Food Addiction

O besity is a growing epidemic in the world today. It is prevalent among adults, but the rate of increase in obesity among children is profoundly worrying. Obesity has contributed to the increased use of aids, which can support weight loss boosters like metabolism. Food is the survival function of any human being. But maybe there are one or more things like candy or chocolates that you like more than two or three times a day. You may not know, but these may be indicators of addiction to food. You may also be addicted to fast food if you have more fast food than usual.

Today's food addiction is like an epidemic. The biggest concern is that many people don't even know that they have a disease and are still over-alimenting. The effect is that a person is addicted to food and consumes a significant number of calories. The explanation that most overweight food consumers do not lose weight is due to their eating habits.

Physicians identify these addicts as people with binge eating disorders. It can lead to severe problems such as diabetes, heart disorders, kidney disorders, and even depression. Food addiction's key symptoms include a constant sense of hunger, shifting in mood, and fluctuation in weight.

Therapy and therapy are the only way to handle the issue of food addiction. You should find a doctor that can help you lose weight in a clinic. If you see a therapist, you can know that you are not the only one with this dilemma that can alleviate the shame. A therapist will help you find out why you are addicted and help you to conquer it with simple methods. He will also teach you how to lose weight healthily.

One must also recognize that it is a long-term process. Hence, patience is essential when you meet with a therapist and a psychologist and must obey their advice appropriately and promptly. Some organizations run rehabilitation services for eating disorders. You can join any of these groups as well. You need to get out of your comfort zone to help yourself deal with the addiction and control your appetite to get rid of unhealthy foods from your diet.

What Foods Are Most Likely to Be Addictive?

The response is frustrating: typically, the most delicious. A researcher involved in food dependency takes stock of the problem in a recent report. His findings suggest that refined, fat, and high glycemic foods are "more commonly correlated with food abuse behavior." Here are several examples:

· Pizza: Pizza is close at the top of the list with its delicious mix of carbs, salt, and fat. "How many spikes ought I to eat?" you ever wondered. The answer: at most, but how to avoid the pizza call. It typically contains more fat per bite than other healthier foods, consisting of many refined ingredients. If you combine all this with salt, you will get a great recipe to get dopamine straight to the next tip. You know it's not essential, but then your brain tells you.

· Treats: Sugar and fat will quickly induce the brain to desire more, candy, cookies, cake, and ice cream. A salty meal is a common practice with a sweet dessert, but it is not a safe option. It allows you to consume sugar and consume more than you need if your food option is unhealthy. Therefore, you can have the extra benefit of calories, fat, and sugar.

· Fried foods: this example is not surprising considering what we already know. Freezes and potato chips are salted and usually fried in oils that do not do your body or brain a lot of good. Although some fried foods are delicious, they are unhealthy and vulnerable to food addiction.

What About Carbonated Drinks?

Soft drinks and fatty and salty foods can be addictive. Research carried out in 2007 found a secure connection between the use of carbonated foods and increased energy intake, that is, the consumption of more calories a day, the existing association between them, and the adverse effects on diet and health well as weight gain. Carbonated beverages were often associated with a decreased consumption of calcium and other nutrients. Consumers of soft drinks are even more at risk for long-term medical issues.

How do carbonated drinks become so addictive? The mystery is straightforward to unwrap: regular carbonated drinks are filled with sugar and often also with caffeine.

Studies show that such beverages can help with weight gain because artificial sweeteners are designed to cause similar reactions in the brain. One research explicitly indicates that individuals who consume artificial sweeteners may have an increased desire for sugar, choose sugar over healthier foods, and be less motivated by health.

Steps to Control Food Addiction
1. Identify the Foods You Are Addicted To

The most addictive foods are rich in sugars, fat, flour, and sodium. Not to mention caffeinated foods such as coffee, soft drinks, and chocolate.

2. Make a Healthy Replacement

When the urge to satisfy your addiction hits, eat another healthier food. When sugar levels drop, hunger hits, instead of consuming sugar, eat healthy protein every 3 or 4 hours, such as cashew or Pará nuts. Eliminate soft drinks (even dietary ones) and industrialized juices (which have a high sugar). Take unsweetened water and natural juices instead.

Some liquids, like orange juice, are very caloric. Prefer to eat the fruit with bagasse.

Don't forget breakfast. It is the most important meal of the day. It must contain fruits, cereals, and protein. When we do not eat breakfast, the desire to eat the food we are addicted to can be uncontrollable.

3. Drink, Instead of Eating

A glass of water may be the solution to what you think is hunger, but which is thirst.

4. Occupy Your Time and Your Mind

Avoid doing nothing when you are not working or studying. The more things you have to do, the less time you'll have to think about food.

5. Practice Physical Exercises

Eating something we like a lot produces a sense of pleasure. Physical activities also provoke such feelings. The difference is that after physical activity, you will feel satisfied and in a good mood, while you will feel sad and guilty when you overeat. Exercising boosts self-esteem and overeating ultimately affects self-esteem.

6. Buy Healthy Foods

When shopping at the supermarket, avoid going through the candy aisles, especially if your object of destruction is in that aisle. Make a list of suitable products for your health and follow them when shopping.

7. Learn or Relearn How to Chew

Chew slowly and thoroughly. Proper chewing produces satiety and good digestion. The stomach sends a satiety message to the brain after 20 minutes from the start of the meal. The more you chew, the longer it will take to eat. You will be sated with a lot less than you think. Therefore, you must allow about 30 minutes to eat your main meals.

8. Seek Expert Advice

Binge eating is a disease, so it needs to be adequately treated. Without the support of a psychologist, nutritionist, and other specialists, you will find it challenging to carry out the treatment until the end. Relapses can be successive, which can be a reason for discouragement and withdrawal.

Overcome Your Food Addiction and Lose Weight!

When you hear the word "addiction," you mostly think of opioids or smoking addiction. They stop little and think about becoming food addicted. You can get addicted as quickly as you can with medicines. Depression plays a significant part, but there are many explanations about why it is possible. Some of the reasons are that you are bored and want to have some food or mental issues you don't know. What would you do if you know you are food-suffering now?

You must first take a deep breath and know it's okay. Don't let panic and anxiety stop you from doing the right thing in your path. Breathe out now. You may want to do it for a couple of seconds before you feel relaxed. You have to focus on thinking before you plan to do something and realize that you can conquer this addiction. The moment you continue to live negatively with food is when you are addicted. Know, "I lose weight, and I'm safe." Don't think about saying, "I should lose weight," even if it's in the present and "now" tense, making it past tense. Now that you are right, the next move should not be such a challenge.

Find a doctor who can help you succeed in a weight loss plan. Joining a program helps you because you're conscious that you're not alone, and you can find out several times what made you addicted to food in the first place. You will be taught a healthier way to lose weight and conquer your addiction by going to a clinic. At first, it might not be convenient, but finally, it is very rewarding.

You should throw out all your fast food while you're doing the plan. This will be a significant change for many. Throwing out the wrong food will build an even better attitude because you know that you can do it for real.

How to Overcome Junk Food Cravings with Weight Loss Hypnosis

1. "Reset" Your Fast Food Attachment

Weight loss hypnotherapy is one of the easiest ways to improve your mindset towards unhealthy food without experiencing excessive cravings or feelings of inadequacy.

For most people, consuming fast food is either an impulsive option or an emotional one. They need to exercise will to stop the momentum, and this process will typically lead to a feeling that they robbed or limited.

You will alter the response mechanism through hypnosis. Ethical behaviors are fun, and the practice improves. You learn to cope well, which means you don't have to rely on food for comfort. Resetting the connection frees your mind and body so that you have fun during weight loss.

2. Get Motivated

The right inspiration will assist you in moving mountains. You have to have the right reasons if you want to get rid of fast food forever.

Most people don't realize that eating nutritious foods benefits their physical wellbeing even more than appearance. By hypnosis of weight loss, people know what the right encouragement is and what important role it plays in the process of weight loss.

Success implies constructive encouragement. You need not confine yourself to discovering the world of balanced eating. You will find it incredibly non-traumatic and even enjoyable if you are enthusiastic about the transition.

3. Get in Touch with Your Emotions

the time or find it challenging to deal with stress in any other way. Contacting inner feelings and unresolved problems will have the power and motivation never to feel the need for fast food.

Have you deemed a compulsive overeater? Were you seen as a fast-food by others? If so, you still have emotional baggage to deal with.

CHAPTER 25:

Eat Healthy and Sleep Better with Hypnosis

Make yourself comfortable.

Find the perfect sleep position.

Inhale through your nose and exhale through your mouth.

Again, inhale through your nose and this time as you exhale, close your eyes.

Repeat this one more time and relax.

Sharpen your breathing focus.

Find stillness in every breath you take, relieve yourself from any tension, and relax.

Let your body relax, soften your heart, quiet your anxious mind, and open to whatever you experience without fighting.

Simply allow your thoughts and experiences to come and go without grasping at them.

Reduce any stress, anxiety, or negative emotions you might have, cool down become deeply and comfortably relaxed.

That's fine.

And as you continue to relax, you can begin the process of reprogramming your mind for your weight loss success because with the right mindset, then you can think positively about what you want to achieve. It begins with changing your mindset and attitude, because the key to losing weight all starts in the mind. One of the very first things you must throw out the window (figuratively) before you start your journey to weight loss is negativity. Negative thinking will just lead you nowhere. It will only pull your moods down, which might trigger emotional eating. Thus, you'll eat more, adding up to that unwanted weight instead of losing it. Remember that you must need to break your old bad habits, and one of them is negative self-talk. You need to change your negative mental views and turn them into positive ones. For example, instead of telling yourself after a few days of workout that nothing is happening or changing, tell yourself that you have done a set of physical activities you have never imagined you can or will do. Make it a point to pat yourself on the back for every little progress you make every day, may it be five additional crunches from what you did yesterday. Understand and accept that this process is a complete transformation, a metamorphosis if you will. This understanding is going to make the process smoother and less painful.

Aside from being positive, you should also be realistic. Don't expect an immediate change in your body. Keep in mind that losing weight is not an overnight thing. It is a long-term process and gradual progress. Set and focus on your goals to keep that negativity at bay.

Don't compare yourself to others, because it will not help you attain your goals in losing weight. First and foremost, keep in mind that each one of us has different body types and compositions. There is a certain diet that may work on you, but not so much for the others. Possibly, some people might need more carbohydrates in their diet, while you might need to drop that and add more protein in your meals. Each one of us is unique. Therefore, your diet plan will surely differ from the person next to you.

Comparing yourself to other people's progress is just a negative thought and will just be unhelpful to you. Remember, always keep a positive outlook and commit to it before you start your diet. For the sake of your long-term success, leave the comparison trap. You're not exactly like the people you idolize, and they're not exactly like you, and that's perfectly fine. Accept that, embrace that and move on with your personal goals.

Be realistic in setting your goals. Think about small and easy to achieve goals that will guide you towards a long term of healthy lifestyle changes. Your goals should be healthy for your body. If you want to truly lose weight and keep it off, it will be a slow uphill battle, with occasional dips and times you'll want to quit. If you expect progress too fast, you will eventually not be able to reach your goals and become discouraged. Don't add extra obstacles for yourself, plan your goals carefully.

If possible, try to find someone who has similar goals as you and work on them together. Two is always better than one and having someone who understands what you are undergoing can be such a relief! An added benefit of having a partner-in-crime (or several) is that you can always hold each other accountable. Accountability is one thing that is easy to start being lax after the first few weeks of a new weight loss program, especially if results aren't quite where you want them to be.

Write down a realistic timetable that you can follow. Start a journal about your daily exercises and meal plan. You can cross out things that you have done already or add new ones along the way. Plot your physical activities. Make time and mark your calendar with daily physical activities. Try to incorporate at least a 15-minute workout on your busy days.

When you become aware of a thought or belief that pins the blame for your extra weight on something outside yourself, if you can find examples of people who've overcome that same cause, realize that it's decision time for you. Choose for yourself whether this is a thought you want to embrace and accept. Does this thought support you living your best life? Does it move you toward your goals, or does it give you an excuse not to go after them?

If you determine your thought no longer serves you, you get to choose another thought instead. Instead of pointing to some external, all-powerful cause for you being overweight, you can choose something different. Track your progress by writing down your step count or workouts daily to keep track of your progress.

Celebrate and embrace your results. Since the path to a healthy lifestyle is mostly hard work and discipline, try to reward yourself for every progress, even if it is small. Treat yourself for a day of pampering, travel to a place you have been wanting to visit, go hiking, have a movie date with friends, or get a new pair of shoes. These kinds of rewards provide you gratification and accomplishments that will make you keep going. Little things do count, and little things also deserve recognition. But keep in mind that your rewards should not compromise your diet plan.

You can also do something like joining an athletic event, a fun run, where you can meet new people that share the same ideals of a healthy lifestyle. You get to learn more about weight loss from others and also share your knowledge. You need to find a source of motivation and keep that source of motivation fresh in your mind, so you don't forget why you embarked on this journey to begin with.

As you focus on your journey of weight loss, keep your stress at bay because too much stress is harmful to the body in many ways, but it also can cause people to gain weight. When the body is under stress, the body will automatically release many hormones and among one of them is cortisol. When the body is under duress and stress, cortisol is released, it can ignite the metabolism for a period of time. However, if the body remains in stressful conditions, the hormone cortisol will continue to be released and actually slow down the metabolism resulting in weight gain.

Everyone experiences stress; there is just no getting around that fact. However, minimizing stressors, as well as learning how to manage the stress in your life will not only help you with losing weight, but it will also make you a more attractive you! High stress in anyone's life often brings out the worst in people. When you are trying to get a man, you want them to see the best of you, not the stressed out you. While you are decreasing your stress level, you will want to increase the amount of sleep you get each night. Lack of sleep is a link to weight gain and because of this, ensuring adequate and appropriate sleep is crucial when trying to lose weight. Sleep is vital for the well-being of the body and the ability for the mind to function, but it is also related to maintaining weight. If you are tired, make sure you sleep, rest or relax, so you are not prone to gaining weight. When a person gets more sleep, the hormone leptin will rise, and when this happens the appetite decreases, which will also decrease body weight.

Gratitude is important in this journey because it teaches you how to make peace with your body, no matter what shape, size or weight it has at the moment. It makes you look at your body with full acceptance and love, saying: "I'm grateful for my body the way it is." It stops you from beating yourself up for being overweight, unhealthy, or out of shape. Be grateful for this learning experience, accept yourself the way you are, and take massive action to get your balance back.

When you express gratitude, you vibrate on a higher energy level, you are positive and happy, and you are simply in a state of satisfaction.

The more things you can find to be grateful for during your weight loss journey, the easier it will be to maintain a positive attitude and keep your motivation up.

It will also get you past those tough moments when you are feeling demotivated to take action and stick to the exercising or eating plan.

This means that you start expressing gratitude for the aspects of your body you would like to have, as if you already have them now. Be grateful for your sexy legs and slim waist. Be grateful for your increased energy levels and strength. Be grateful for the ability to wear smaller clothes. You get the drill. Feel the positive energy of gratitude flowing through your body as you imagine these things are true. By going through this exercise you'll notice the positive change in your thought patterns.

With the level of personal growth you will achieve and the habits you will change in this session of hypnosis, you will feel like a completely different person. You will have more power, self–confidence, and love yourself more than you ever thought possible before. That's a change from the inside out. That's what lasts. And, at the end of the day, that's what truly matters.

Take a deep breath and allow your breath to return its natural rate as you return to your normal consciousness.

As you continue to breathe, note that, right now, at this moment, you have no worries. You are just a relaxed body. Any distractions that arise while you tell yourself this can wait.

Repeat the following phrases:

- I am relaxed

- I am balanced

- I can deal with any worries later

- I am relaxed

- I am balanced

The whole earth supports you in your relaxation and balance. Feel yourself supported and held.

Feel that everything you have done in your life has brought you to this moment without errors or mistakes.

This moment is perfect.

CHAPTER 26:

Deep Relaxing techniques

Since we have seen that emotions are the first obstacle to a healthy and correct relationship with food, we are going to look specifically at the most suitable techniques to appease them. Not only is that, these techniques very important to make hypnosis deeply effective in order to achieve the desired goals.

In fact, autogenic training is one of the techniques of self-hypnosis. What does self-hypnosis mean? As the word suggests, it is a form of self-induced hypnosis. Beyond the various techniques available, all have the objective of concentrating a single thought object. To say it seems easy, but it is incredible how, in reality, our mind is constantly distracted and even overlaps distant thoughts between them. This leads to emotional tension with repercussions in everyday life.

Other self-hypnosis techniques that we will not deal with in-depth include Benson's and Erickson's.

Benson's is inspired by oriental transcendental meditation. It is based on the constant repetition of a concept in order to favor a great concentration. Specifically, he recommends repeating the word that evokes the concept several times. It is the easiest and fastest technique ever. It really takes 10-15 minutes a day. Just because it's so simple doesn't mean it's not effective. And you will also need to familiarize yourself with it. Especially for those who are beginners with self-hypnosis. In fact, this could be the first technique to try right away to approach this type of practice.

You sit with your eyes closed in a quiet room and focus on breathing and relax the muscles. Therefore continually think about the object of meditation. If your thought turns away, bring it back to the object. To be sure to practice this self-hypnosis for at least 10 minutes, just set a timer.

Erickson's is apparently more complex. The first step involves creating a new self-image that you would like to achieve. So we start from something we don't like about ourselves and mentally create the positive image that we would like to create.

In our specific case, we could start from the idea of us being overweight and transform that idea into an image of us in perfect shape, satisfied with ourselves in front of the mirror.

Then we focus on three objects around the subject, then three noises, and finally three sensations. It takes little time to concentrate on these things. Gradually decrease this number. Therefore 2 objects, 2 noises, and 2 sensations. Better if the objects are small and bright and unusual sensations, which are hardly paid attention. For example, the feeling of the shirt that we wear in contact with our skin. You get to one, and then you leave your mind wandering. We take the negative image we have and calmly transform it mentally into the positive one. At the end of this practice, you will feel great energy and motivation.

Autogenic Training

Autogenic training is a highly effective self-induced relaxation technique without external help. It is called "training" because it includes a series of exercises that allow the gradual and passive acquisition of changes in muscle tone, vascular function, cardiac and pulmonary activity, neurovegetative balance, and state of consciousness. But don't be frightened by this word. His exercises do not require a particular theoretical preparation nor a radical modification of one's habits. Practicing this activity allows you to live a profound and repeatable experience at all times.

Autogenic means "self-generating," unlike hypnosis and self-hypnosis, which are actively induced by an operator or the person himself.

In essence, the goal is to achieve inner harmony so that we can best face the difficulties of everyday life. It is a complementary tool to hypnosis. The two activities are intertwined. Practicing both of them allows for a better overall experience. In fact, hypnosis helps well to act directly on the subconscious. But in order for hypnosis to be effective, it is necessary to have already prepared an inner calm such that there is no resistance to the instructions given by the hypnotherapist. The origins of autogenic training are rooted in the activity of hypnosis. In the latter, there is an exclusive relationship between hypnotist and hypnotized. Those who are hypnotized must, therefore, be in a state of maximum receptivity in order to be able to reach a state of constructive passivity in order to create the ideal relationship with the hypnotist.

Those who approach autogenic training and have already undergone hypnosis sessions can deduce the main training guidelines from the principles of hypnosis. The difference is that you become your own hypnotist. You must, therefore, assume an attitude of receptive availability towards you. Such activity also allows a higher spiritual introspection, feeling masters of one's emotional state. This undoubtedly brings countless advantages in everyday life.

So I usually suggest everyone try a hypnosis session and then do a few days of autogenic training before they start using hypnosis again on a daily basis. It's the easiest way to approach the relaxation techniques on your own and start to become familiar with the psycho-physical sensations given by these practices. Mine is a spontaneous suggestion. If you have tried meditation and relaxation techniques in the past, you can also go directly into guided hypnosis. In any case, autogenic training can be useful regardless of the level of familiarity with these practices.

It is clear that if you have little time in your days, it makes no sense to put so much meat on the fire. Let's remember that they are still relaxation techniques. If we see them too much as "training," we could associate obligations and bad emotions that go against the principle of maximum relaxation. So I'm not saying do autogenic training and hypnosis every day, 10 push-ups, crunches, and maybe yoga, and then you will be relaxed and at peace with your body. This approach is not good. It is about finding your balance and harmony in a practice that has to be pleasant and deliberate.

Basic Autogenic Training Exercises

The basic exercises of the A.T. are classically divided into 6 exercises, of which 2 fundamental and 4 complementary. Before the 6 exercises, you practice an induction to calm and relaxation, while at the end a recovery and then awakening.

These exercises are considered as consecutive phases to be carried out in each session. It is not mandatory to carry out all the steps together. Especially initially each exercise will have to be understood individually. But if you intend to stop, for example, in the fourth exercise and not do all of them, you will necessarily have to do the other 3 exercises in the same session first. The duration of the session remains unchanged, however, because when you add exercises, you will make each phase last less.

First exercise - "The heaviness." It s a very useful exercise to overcome psychophysical problems related to muscular tensions that derive from emotional tensions.

Second exercise - "The heat." It serves to relieve circulatory problems, in all cases where there is a problem of reduced blood flow to the extremities.

Third exercise - "The heart." It is a highly suggestive exercise that allows you to regain contact with that part of the body that we traditionally deal with emotions.

Fourth exercise - "The breath." It produces a better oxygenation of the blood and organs.

Fifth exercise - The solar plexus. It helps a lot of those who suffer from digestive problems.

Sixth exercise - The Fresh Forehead. Produces a brain constriction vessel that can be very useful to reduce headaches, especially if linked to physical or mental overload.

Recommended Positions

The following positions are suitable for both autogenic training and hypnosis and relaxation techniques in general. I suggest initially to use the lying down position and to use it later in hypnosis for virtual gastric bandaging in order to simulate the position on the surgical couch.

Lie Down

This position, at least at the beginning, is the most used for its comfort. You lie on your back (face up) and your legs slightly apart with your toes out. The arms are slightly detached from the torso and are slightly bent. The fingers are detached from each other and slightly arched.

On the Armchair

You sit with a chair attached to the wall. Your back is firmly against the backrest, and your head rests against the wall. You can place a cushion between your head and the wall.

Alternatively, you can use a high chair to rest your head-on. The feet should be flat firmly on the floor, with a 90-degree angle on the legs.

The tips of the feet should be placed on the outside. The arms should be resting on the supports (where present) or on the thighs.

If there are supports, the hands should be left dangling.

If they are not present, the hands are resting on the legs, and the fingers are separate.

Position of the Coachman

This position allows you to be seated but without particular basic support. It can be practiced wherever you have something to sit on (a chair, a stone, a stool...).

You sit, for example, on the chair very far forward without leaning forward with your back.

Your feet must be flat firmly on the ground, with the tips pointing outwards. Your back should bend forward by resting your forearms on your thighs and letting your hands dangle between your legs so that they do not touch each other. Pivot your neck forward as much as possible, and relax your shoulders and jaw.

Other Suggestions

To achieve the best results, the environment must be quiet, the phone and any form of technological distraction must be disconnected beforehand. In the room, there must be a very soft light with a constant temperature that allows neither hot nor cold. The environmental conditions, in fact, influence our mood, and the acquisition of a correct position guarantees an objective relaxation of all the muscles.

Do not wear clothes that tighten and restrict your movement: for this purpose also remove the watch and glasses and loosen the belt.

It goes without saying that constancy is very important for achieving a psychic balance. It only takes 10 minutes a day, but a real reluctance is to be taken into consideration. Before doing this practice, you really need to give yourself some time. It must be a deliberate practice. This is one of the reasons why it is not advisable to practice it in small time gaps between commitments, but rather in dedicated time slots.

Also, it is advisable not to practice the exercises immediately after lunch to avoid sleep. At the end of each workout, perform awakening exercises except for the evening just before going to sleep.

At first, checking the relaxation of the various parts of the body will require some reflection. But over time and practice, everything will become more instinctive. Do not expect great results in the first days of practice. Do not abandon the practice immediately because, like anything else, you cannot expect to know how to do it immediately.

One last tip is to not be too picky when it comes to checking the position to take. In fact, the indications provided are broad; it is not necessary to interpret them rigidly.

Conclusion

Congratulations! You've now learned the basics of gastric band hypnosis and how to use it to empower yourself and strengthen the confidence in your ability to change habits and lose weight. Aside from biological and environmental, many psychological influences shape your thoughts, feelings, and behavioral patterns when it comes to eating.

Most people claim that weight loss hypnosis is a simple way to solve weight issues. People are also attracted by hypnosis because they feel they don't have to do any workouts, they can eat whatever they want, and all they have to do is close their eyes and lose weight in minutes. That's just not true.

No magic pills are available to lose weight, be it by hypnosis or some other form of weight loss. It is not possible to lose weight immediately after only one hypnosis session. A well-trained and professional hypnotist takes many sessions to achieve the best possible outcomes.

Several websites on the Internet say that weight loss hypnosis will produce dramatic results after just one session. Most people are likely to be insulted by this argument because everybody knows it is not possible to lose the weight overnight-however successful the hypnotist is.

Practicing weight loss hypnosis was another method for those who want to shape their bodies as they wish. There are also men who don't like their own body image. This leads to a loss of self-esteem and confidence. Some people prefer to use workouts and other lifestyle strategies to achieve their ideal body shape. Unfortunately, few tests are churning out. That is why people who understood the technique of mental strength resort to hypnosis to lose their body mass. You will find an absolute guide on how to use that method to attain the correct body shape on the internet. It is up to you to use your brain's strength to understand how useful it can be for you.

Hypnotizing is generally known to remove the inner self concentration. It generally happens in the same way as in a trance. Slimming hypnosis is an operation performed with the aid of the hypnotherapist. In this case, the person who wants to slightly repeat the messages given to him in the form of sentences, phrases, or even pictures may do so verbally. Mental images often play a major role in achieving the same result.

One thing you must remember is that your mind needs to concentrate more as you go through the hypnotizing process. In certain states, the mind and the subconscious state are very sensitive. You are well-positioned to react suggestively to the circumstances which lead you to your ideal body so that the best results can be obtained in a very short period of time. It is an activity that many people can do effectively with much less effort.

The research centers and interested stakeholders have performed many studies. Research has shown that people typically achieve fair outcomes using this form of hypnosis. This method can also lose up to an average of 2.7 kilograms.

Hypnotized, however, does not always function well on its own. You will take into account other behaviors that can effectively improve your weight loss. Take the best diet plan with your nutritionist's support. Not just this, you should do the workouts that will reduce your excess weight. In addition, you will try to follow a balanced lifestyle, which would help you in the end. Regulate your sleep hours, for example, and avoid any bad habits. If you use this routine and use all the tricks, you get the best performance. Ultimately, you learn to regulate your mind to lose weight. You train your subconscious mind to decrease your body mass, and if you practice this cycle, it will happen.

CPSIA information can be obtained
at www.ICGtesting.com
Printed in the USA
BVHW011555200221
600497BV00025B/9